MCQs in Pedodontics with Explanations for PG Dental Entrance Examinations

MCQs in Pedodontics with Explanations for PG Dental Entrance Examinations

Also for BDS & MDS Professional Examinations

Satish Chandra

Best Teacher Awardee
Ex-Member, Dental Council of India
Ex-Director and Professor
Sardar Patel Institute of Dental and Medical Sciences, Lucknow
Ex-Professor and Head of the Department and Dean
Dental Faculty, UP KG University of Dental Sciences (Formerly KG Medical College, CSM Medical University and KG Medical University, Lucknow)
Ex-Professor, Dean, Head and Principal
DJ College of Dental Sciences and Research, Modinagar, UP
Ex-Professor, Dean, Head and Principal, Institute of Dental Sciences, Bareilly
Ex-Principal, Professor and Head of the Department, Awadh Institute of Dental Sciences, Lucknow
Paper Setter and Examiner for BDS, MDS and PGME Examinations in Many Universities
Ex-Member, Dental Council of India

Shaleen Chandra

Professor and Head of the Dept., Saraswati Dental College and Hospital, 233 Tiwariganj, Faizabad Road, Juggour, Lucknow
Ex-Professor and Head of the Dept., Sardar Patel Institute of Dental and Medical Sciences, Lucknow
Ex-Assistant Professor, Rama Dental College and Hospital and Research Centre, Kanpur
Ex-Lecturer, UP KG University of Dental Sciences (Formerly KG Medical College, CSM Medical University and KG Medical University), Lucknow
Ex-Lecturer, Buddha Institute of Dental Sciences, Kankar Bagh, Patna
Paper Setter and Examiner of BDS, MDS and PGME Examinations in Many Universities

Girish Chandra

Rajendra Nagar Dental Clinic, Lucknow

JAYPEE BROTHERS
MEDICAL PUBLISHERS (P) LTD
New Delhi

Published by

Jitendar P Vij
Jaypee Brothers Medical Publishers (P) Ltd
EMCA House, 23/23B Ansari Road, Daryaganj, **New Delhi** 110 002, India
Phones: +91-11-23272143, +91-11-23272703,
+91-11-23282021, +91-11-23245672
Fax: +91-11-23276490, +91-11-23245683
e-mail: jaypee@jaypeebrothers.com
Visit our website: www.jaypeebrothers.com

Branches

- 2/B, Akruti Society, Jodhpur Gam Road Satellite
Ahmedabad 380015, Phones: +91-079-30988717, +91-079-26926233
e-mail: jpamdvd@rediffmail.com
- 202 Batavia Chambers, 8 Kumara Krupa Road, Kumara Park East
Bangalore 560 001, Phones: +91-80-22285971, +91-80-22382956,
+91-80-30614073 Tele Fax : +91-80-22281761
e-mail: jaypeemedpubbgal@eth.net
- 282 IIIrd Floor, Khaleel Shirazi Estate, Fountain Plaza, Pantheon Road
Chennai 600 008, Phones: +91-44-28262665, +91-44-28269897 Fax: +91-44-28262331
e-mail: jpchen@eth.net
- 4-2-1067/1-3, Ist Floor, Balaji Building, Ramkote Cross Road
Hyderabad 500 095, Phones: +91-40-55610020, +91-40-24758498, +91-40-30940929
Fax: +91-40-24758499
e-mail: jpmedpub@rediffmail.com
- 1A Indian Mirror Street, Wellington Square
Kolkata 700 013, Phones: +91-33-22456075, +91-33-22451926, +91-33-30901926
Fax: +91-33-22456075 e-mail: jpbcal@cal.vsnl.net.in
- 106 Amit Industrial Estate, 61 Dr SS Rao Road, Near MGM Hospital Parel
Mumbai 400 012, Phones: +91-22-24124863, +91-22-24104532
+91-22-30926896 Fax: +91-22-24160828
e-mail: jpmedpub@bom7.vsnl.net.in
- "KAMALPUSHPA" 38, Reshimbag, Opp. Mohota Science College, Umred Road
Nagpur 440 009 (MS), Phones: +91-712-3945220, + 91-712-2704275
Fax: +91-712-2704275 e-mail: jpmednagpur @rediffmail.com

MCQs in Pedodontics

First Edition: **2006**

ISBN 81-8061-804-8

Typeset at JPBMP typesetting unit
Printed at Gopsons Papers Ltd., A-14, Sector 60, Noida

Preface

This book is written keeping professional and PG Dental Entrance Examinations in mind. Explanations have been given with the answers. It is based on the experience of many toppers regarding flying success in the examinations. This book will guide in preparations for examination. The questions in this book have been compiled after analyzing many question papers of previous years.

The secret of success in competitive examination lies in proper guidance and hard work. This book simplifies your preparation by making you work more efficiently. For the sake of convenience we have written four MCQs books namely: *MCQs in Pedodontics, MCQs in Operative Dentistry and Endodontics, MCQs in Oral and Maxillofacial Surgery and MCQs in Periodontics*, which have been divided subjectwise, one book on each major subject. Some allied subjects have been joined together. All the books on MCQs will be true friends and a great asset for the candidates of dental professional examinations, the postgraduate dental entrance examinations and interview, and also for practitioners. The trend is very fast changing toward MCQs. These books will also be very useful for graduate and postgraduate courses, as these contain questions, which are likely to be asked in periodical assessments during graduate and postgraduate courses and in final examinations.

For the preparation for examinations the aim of these books is to encourage the readers to detect areas of weakness in understanding the subject matter so that they may again study the textbooks for better and comprehensive review of the subject.

Every effort has been made to update all the books. All the books will be very useful for all the students and will prepare them to face any examination with full confidence.

Satish Chandra
Shaleen Chandra
Girish Chandra

Tips for Success

1. Start your preparations at least one year in advance. Give six months for initial preparation (Reading Textbooks and solving MCQs), 4 months for final preparation (Solving MCQs from books) and last two months for revision of MCQs.
2. Procure all study material and finish subject by subject.
3. Plan your study hours.
4. Consult your seniors who have passed the examinations with a good score. Follow their advice but not blindly.
5. Read the textbook of the subjects thoroughly from the beginning to the end. Do not do selective reading except only in revision.
6. Be organised in your study.
7. Aim for the top because you will invariably fall short.
8. Practice self-assessment tests and solve model test papers to know which chapters require revision and to get a feel of examination conditions.
9. Understand each chapter of each subject and attempt connected MCQs before proceeding to the next chapter. If you correctly answer less than 90% of MCQs, repeat the chapter.
10. Practise, practise and practise MCQs again and again with reasoning.
11. Time yourself while solving model test papers and examination question papers.
12. Relax and be tension-free while attempting questions in the examination.
13. Read the questions carefully to understand them, think and then answer.

Information and Suggestions

Remember

- You can do it. Always try for the top slots because if you aim for the sky, you would at least reach the hilltop.
- You can do it and have to do it.

Tentative dates of various entrance exams			*Approximate no.of seats available*
All India PG	-	Jan	130
AIIMS	-	Jan/June	4
BHU	-	June	2
PGI Chandigarh	-	June/Nov	4
MAHE	-	May	50
Various state/ College/ University entrances	-	Jan to Dec	1000

The following is the approximate percentage of MCQs appeared in the various postgraduate entrance in previous years.

Subject	*No. of MCQs %age*	*Weeks required for revision*	
		Textbooks	*MCQs books*
1. Purely Preclinical	3	1	1
2. Applied Preclinical	8	2	2
3. Oral and Dental Pathology & Oral Medicine	25	5	5
4. Oral and Maxillofacial Surgery	9	2	2
5. Periodontics	5	1	1
6. Prosthodontics & Applied Dental Material	14	3	3
7. Conservative Dentistry	8	2	2
8. Orthodontics	8	2	2
9. Dental Radiology	3	2	2
10. Endodontics	5	2	2
11. Community Dentistry	2	1	1

Contd...

Contd...

Subject	No. of MCQs %age	Weeks required for revision	
		Textbooks	MCQs books
12. Gen. Medicine and Surgery	5	1	1
13. Pedodontics and Preventive Dentistry	5	1	1
Total	100	25	27

1. Only hard labor and vast knowledge are not enough but mastering the technique of taking MCQs examination is equally important.
2. First clear the basic fundamentals to have wider and better understanding of the subject. You must read the textbooks as much as possible.
3. Do not attempt the questions that you are not sure of. Negative marks due to guesswork always take you down in the merit list. Even 1 mark can change your merit tremendously.
4. It is better to leave a question rather than to attempt it wrongly.
5. Research in psychology has concluded that most of us mark the right choice first and due to second thoughts mark a wrong choice.
6. The entrance examinations are to test the basic fundamental knowledge of the subject. Mostly the choices are straight forward and not to trick you. Answer each question from general principles rather than from exceptions.
7. Appear in all the entrance examinations in which you are eligible. You never know when luck may favor you.

Contents

1

Introduction, Rationale, Objective, Scope and Future of Pedodontics

1. Pedodontics involves treatment of patients:

A. Up to the age of 15 years

B. Up to the age of 12 years

C. Up to the age of 18 years

D. Up to the age of 16 years

Answer

1.A. Pedodontics or pediatric dentistry is an age-related specialty, meant for preventive and curative dental and oral health care of infants and children, usually upto the age of 15 years.

2

General Concepts of Growth and Development

1. **The primary teeth begin to calcify:**
   - A. Between eight to twelve weeks of fetal life
   - B. Between six to seven months of fetal life
   - C. Between four to six weeks of fetal life
   - D. Between four to six months of fetal life

2. **Ectodermal cells are responsible for:**
   - A. Pulp formation
   - B. Cementum formation
   - C. Periodontal tissue formation
   - D. Determining shape of crown and root

3. **In the average child, teeth generally in the process of calcification at birth are:**
   - A. The deciduous anterior, canines and first primary molars only
   - B. All primary teeth and first permanent molars
   - C. All primary teeth only
   - D. All primary teeth and some permanent teeth

4. **Which branchial arch is known as Hyoid's arch:**
   - A. First branchial arch
   - B. Second branchial arch
   - C. Third branchial arch
   - D. Fourth branchial arch

5. **Which branchial arch disappears?**
   - A. 3rd
   - B. 4th
   - C. 5th
   - D. 6th

6. Third ear ossicle is derived from:
A. 1st branchial arch
B. 2nd branchial arch
C. 3rd branchial arch
D. 4th branchial arch

7. Permanent teeth begin their eruption into the oral cavity when:
A. 1/4th of their roots are formed
B. 1/2th of their roots are formed
C. 3/4th of their roots are formed
D. 4/5th of their roots are formed

Answers

1.D. Calcification begins first in central incisor, i.e. between 13 to 16 weeks in utero and lastly in second molar, i.e. between 16 to 24 weeks in utero.

2.D. Individual tooth germs are influenced by epigenetic factors to assume their characteristic shapes and sizes in the dental arches. Enamel of teeth is derived from ectoderm and the mesoderm provides the anlagen for the dentin, pulp and periodontal formation.

3.D. Calcification occurs by the precipitation of inorganic calcium salts within the deposited matrix. Dates for third molars are not definite hence not accounted for.

4.B. Second branchial arch is the precursor of a third ear ossicle, the stapes. It also contributes to small portions of the malleus and incus.

5.C. Fifth branchial arch is a transitory structure and disappears almost as soon as it is formed.

6.B. Branchial arches appear at approximately 24 to 26 days of intrauterine life.

7.C. The time interval between crown completion and beginning of eruption until the tooth is in full occlusion is approximately 3 to 5 years for permanent teeth.

3

Dentition: Its Development and Speech

1. **The congenital absence of tooth is attributable to which stage of tooth development?**
   A. Initiation and proliferation
   B. Histodifferentiation
   C. Morphodifferentiation
   D. Apposition

2. **The permanent teeth have all the following characteristics as compared to the deciduous teeth *except*:**
   A. More prominent pulp horns
   B. Larger occlusal table
   C. More pronounced contact points
   D. Less vascular pulp

3. **The relative size of the pulp chambers to the crown in permanent and deciduous teeth is:**
   A. Smaller in permanent teeth
   B. Smaller in deciduous teeth
   C. Same in both
   D. None of the above

4. **Anodontia occurs when there is defective:**
   A. Initiation stage
   B. Mineralization stage
   C. Histodifferentiation stage
   D. Morphodifferentiation stage

5. **The growth stages of tooth development include the following:**
   A. Initiation
   B. Proliferation
   C. Histodifferentiation
   D. All of the above

6. **The usual eruption sequence in the deciduous dentition is as follows:**
   A. Canines, lateral incisors, central incisors, first molars, second molars
   B. Lateral incisors, central incisors, first molars, canines, second molars
   C. Central incisors, canines, lateral incisors, first molars, second molars
   D. Central incisors, lateral incisors, first molars, canines, second molars

7. **Usual eruption sequence of permanent maxillary teeth is:**
   A. Central incisor, lateral incisor, canine, first premolar, second premolar, I molar and II molar
   B. I molar, central incisor, lateral incisor, first premolar, second premolar, canine, second molar, third molar
   C. I molar, central incisor, lateral incisor, canine, I premolar II premolar, I molar, II molar and III molar
   D. I molar, II molar, central incisor, lateral incisor, canine, I premolar, II premolar, III molar

8. **Usual eruption sequence of permanent mandibular teeth is:**
   A. Central incisor, lateral incisor, canine, I premolar, II premolar, I molar, II molar, III molar
   B. Lateral incisor, central incisor, canine, II premolar, I premolar, I molar, II molar, III molar
   C. I molar, central incisor, lateral incisor, canine, I premolar, II premolar, II molar and III molar
   D. I molar, II molar, lateral incisor, central incisor, canine, I premolar, II premolar, II molar

9. **At 8 years of age how many deciduous teeth are present mesial to first permanent molar?**
   A. Two　　B. Five
   C. Four　　D. Three

10. **At 8 years of age which permanent tooth is erupting?**
   A. The first molar
   B. The first bicuspid
   C. The lateral incisor
   D. The cuspid

11. The first deciduous tooth to erupt is the:
A. Maxillary lateral incisor
B. Mandibular central incisor
C. Mandibular lateral incisor
D. Maxillary central incisor

12. Most primary arches have the following shape:
A. Ovoid B. Square
C. Triangular D. Hexagonal

13. The roots of primary molars are:
A. Relatively shorter than roots of permanent teeth
B. Relatively longer than roots of permanent teeth
C. Shorter than roots of anterior teeth
D. Longer than roots of permanent teeth

14. The last deciduous tooth to be replaced by a permanent tooth is usually the:
A. Mandibular canine
B. Maxillary canine
C. Mandibular second molar
D. Maxillary second molar

15. An important morphologic difference in deciduous teeth that necessitates a modification of one of Black's principles is that:
A. The occlusal surface does not have pits or fissures
B. The crown is bell-shaped
C. Secondary dentin does not form
D. Occlusal enamel is thicker than the proximal enamel

16. How do the widths of second primary molar and its successor compare:
A. Depends upon the tooth size in relation to jaw size
B. About the same
C. Successor is wider
D. Primary molar is wider

17. If a child loses his primary molars at or before 5 years of age:
A. The eruption of premolars will be delayed
B. The eruption of premolars will be accelerated
C. No effect
D. Cannot say

18. In the gingival one-third of the deciduous molars, enamel rods, as they travel to outer surface are:
A. Inclined occlusally
B. Inclined gingivally
C. Parallel
D. None of the above

19. Out of the followings the last tooth which erupts into the oral cavity is:
A. Maxillary canine
B. Maxillary 1st premolar
C. Maxillary 2nd premolar
D. Mandibular 2nd premolar

20. How many roots does a primary maxillary first molar have?
A. One **B.** Two
C. Three **D.** Four

Answers

1.A. Problems during the initiation and proliferation stages are known to produce dental anomalies in both number and structure.

2.A. Deciduous teeth have more prominent pulp horns. Especially the mesial horns of deciduous teeth are relatively higher than those of the permanent teeth.

3.A. Pulp chambers of deciduous teeth are larger due to thinner dentin walls.

4.A. Anodontia is the absence of teeth. It may be total (complete) and partial (incomplete). This is more common in the permanent dentition.

5.D. Initiation is also known as Bud stage, proliferation is known as cap stage and histodifferentiation as Bell stage.

6.D. Indications that teeth are going to erupt are (i) increased salivation (ii) increased finger sucking, (iii) day time restlessness, (iv) rubbing of the gums, and (v) reduced appetite.

7.B. The time interval between crown completion and beginning of eruption until the tooth is in full occlusion is approximately 3 to 5 years for permanent teeth.

8.C. Canine erupts earlier in mandibular arch as compared to maxillary arch.

9.D. Deciduous canine, first molar and second molar are present mesial to first permanent molar at 8 years of age.

10.C. Lateral incisor erupts between the age of 7 and 8 years.

11.B. Deciduous mandibular central incisor erupts at the age of 6 months.

12.A. Most primary arches have ovoid shape.

13.A. The roots of deciduous molars, in order to accommodate bud of permanent tooth, are more flared than the roots of permanent molars.

14.D. Eruption age of permanent maxillary canine is between 11 and 12 years

15.B. The deciduous teeth have wider crown mesiodistally than they are occlusocervically. Hence, they appear more bulbous than permanent teeth.

16.D. Buccolingually, the deciduous molars have narrower occlusal table than permanent molars.

17.A. If loss occurs at the age of 8,9 and 10 years, then the eruption of premolars will be greatly accelerated.

18.A. In the gingival one-third of the permanent molars, enamel rods as they travel to outer surface are inclined gingivally.

19.A. Eruption age of permanent maxillary canine is between 11 and 12 years.

20.C. Primary maxillary first molar has three roots, i.e. mesiobuccal, distobuccal and palatal.

4

Developmental Disturbances in Dentition and Surrounding Structures

1. **Neonatal tooth is the:**
   A. Tooth which erupted soon after birth
   B. Tooth which erupted in between 0 and 30 days after birth
   C. Tooth present at birth
   D. Tooth which erupts at 6 months of age

2. **When two teeth are joined only at the cementum it is known as:**
   A. Dilaceration
   B. Concrescence
   C. Gemination
   D. Fusion

3. **The most common congenitally missing permanent tooth in the maxillary arch leaving the third molar is:**
   A. Second molar
   B. Second premolar
   C. Central incisor
   D. Lateral incisor

4. **Enamel infarction is:**
   A. Hypoplasia B. Hyperplasia
   C. Minute crack D. Discoloration

5. **A rare congenital syndrome characterized by absence of clavicles, enlarged fontanels, open head sutures, delayed development of dentition is known as:**
   A. Osteodentin dysplasia
   B. Marie-Sainton syndrome
   C. Cleidocranial dysostosis
   D. All of the above

6. **The primary teeth which are most often ankylosed are:**
   A. Maxillary canines
   B. Mandibular canine
   C. Maxillary second molar
   D. Mandibular second molar

7. **Dentinogenesis imperfecta differs from amelogenesis imperfecta as the former is:**
   A. Characterized by brown colored spots on the enamel
   B. Characterized by calcification of pulp chambers and the root canals of the teeth
   C. Due to formation of faulty enamel matrix
   D. A hereditary disturbance

8. **Amelogenesis imperfecta can affect:**
   A. Deciduous teeth only
   B. Permanent teeth only
   C. Deciduous and permanent teeth
   D. Periodontium

9. **Disturbances in the morphodifferentiation stage of the tooth germ results in:**
   A. Ameloblastoma
   B. Abnormal forma and size of teeth
   C. Abnormal location of teeth
   D. Abnormal number of teeth

10. **Accepted latency period between exfoliation of deciduous teeth and eruption of succedaneous permanent tooth is:**
    A. 3 months B. 6 months
    C. 9 months D. 12 months

11. **A primary second molar becomes ankylosed most commonly:**
    A. During root formation
    B. During physiological root resorption
    C. Due to failure of alveolar bone of tooth to grow
    D. All of the above

Answers

1.B. Teeth present at birth are known as natal teeth.

2.B. Concrescence of teeth is actually a form of fusion that occurs after root formation has been completed. The teeth are united by cementum only.

3.D. The most common missing permanent tooth is the third molar.

4.C. Due to fall or blow from a hard object, minute cracks (crazing) of the enamel of the anterior teeth occurs.

5.C. In the anterior region, unerupted supernumerary teeth may be present. Deciduous teeth are retained and permanent teeth unerupted.

6.D. If ankylosed anterior primary teeth are causing delay in eruption of the permanent tooth, it should be removed.

7.B. Amelogenesis imperfecta is an ectodermal defect and thus mesodermal structures of the tooth, like dentin and pulp, are always found normal.

8.C. Amelogenesis imperfecta can affect both the deciduous as well as the permanent dentition. The color of the teeth is usually chalky-white but sometimes it is yellow or even dark brown.

9.B. In morphodifferentiation stage, the shape and size of a tooth is determined. Any disturbance in this stage will result in abnormal forms and sizes of teeth, e.g. microdontia and macrodontia.

10.B. The time interval between crown completion and beginning of eruption until the tooth is in full occlusion is approximately 3 to 5 years for permanent teeth.

11.B. Invasion of the osteoclastic cells takes place due to the inflammation and injury to the periodontal ligament which causes irregular resorption of the root surface. After resorption when repair takes place, mechanical lock or fusion takes place between alveolar bone and root surface.

5

Importance of First Permanent Molar

1. **The extraction of the upper first molar may be indicated:**
   - **A.** To provide space for eruption of second molar
   - **B.** When second premolar is palatally placed
   - **C.** When it is rotated
   - **D.** When its prognosis is very poor

Answer

1.D. The first permanent molar is a very important tooth, from functional and developmental point of views.

6

Diagnostic Devices and Treatment Planning in Pedodontics

1. **An occluded submandibular duct is best demonstrated by:**
   A. Cephalograms
   B. Percussion
   C. Occlusal radiographs
   D. Sialograms

2. **The following should be undertaken to reduce the child's exposure to X-rays:**
   A. Decrease the tube to teeth distance
   B. Use fast films
   C. Use slow films
   D. Increase the tube to teeth distance

3. **Which of the following is of greatest help in diagnosing ankylosis of a deciduous first molar?**
   A. Solid metallic sound on percussion
   B. Cushioned sound on percussion
   C. Loss of vitality on electric pulp test
   D. Radiographic density of lamina dura

4. **Standard size of an I.O.P.A. X-ray film is:**
   A. 22 × 35 mm B. 24 × 40 mm
   C. 32 × 41 mm D. 25 × 40 mm

5. **Most common size of occlusal X-ray film is:**
   A. 50 × 75 mm B. 45 × 75 mm
   C. 60 × 78 mm D. 57 × 76 mm

6. **X-ray film is relatively insensitive to:**
   A. White light
   B. Blue and green light
   C. Red light
   D. Yellow and red light

Answers

1.D. Sialography is the radiological examination of salivary glands and their ducts after injection of a radiopaque medium into the gland substance via the duct opening.

2.B. Young, rapidly growing tissue in children is more radiosensitive as compared to the mature tissue in adults.

3.D. If ankylosis takes place, the tooth remains fixed in relation to the adjacent teeth and structures, and the periodontal membrane of the tooth is interrupted.

4.C. I.O.P.A films are found in three sizes

Size 0 (for children) –22 × 35 mm

Size 1 (for adult-anterior teeth) –24 × 40 mm

Size 2 (standard size) –32 × 41 mm

5.D. It is used to take the occlusal view X-ray of the entire arch. It gives idea that a lesion is present lingually or facially, and about the size of the lesion.

6.D. The areas potentially at risk from dental radiography are eyes, bone marrow in jaws and thyroid gland.

7

Pedodontic Practice, Child Behavior and Management of Anxiety and Pain

1. **Unpremedicated children should not be kept in the dental chair for period longer than:**
   A. Ninety minutes
   B. One hour
   C. Fifteen minutes
   D. Half an hour

2. **Bribery for the child dental patient should:**
   A. Never be utilized because it rarely accomplishes any good
   B. Always be utilized
   C. Never be used to induce good behavior
   D. None of the above

3. **Introjection is the:**
   A. Rejection of a bad object
   B. Rejection of a good object
   C. Attempt by child to take into his/her mouth a good object
   D. Attempt by child to take a bad object into the mouth

4. **Projection is the:**
   A. Rejection of a good object
   B. Attempt to take a good object into the mouth
   C. Rejection of a bad object from the mouth
   D. Attempt to take a bad object into the mouth

5. **The anterior teeth of both dentitions:**
   A. Serve for growth and development of the jaws
   B. Are not an important psychologic factor for well being of the individual
   C. Are a primary factor in the psychologic well being of the individual
   D. Serve for incision only

6. In managing an eight years old child the dentist should keep in mind that a child of this age is:
A. Generally uncooperative
B. Prone to separation anxiety
C. Extremely afraid of strangers
D. Susceptible to praise

7. How should toys be used in child management ?
A. Gift
B. Bribe
C. Reward
D. All of the above are correct

8. Behavioral management in a child can be done by:
A. Positive approach
B. Team attitude
C. Organization
D. All of the above

9. Which of the following statements is correct?
A. Highly anxious parents affect their child's behavior negatively below 4 years of age
B. Children who enjoyed their past medical experiences positively are more likely to be cooperative
C. Both of the above
D. None

10. Which of the following responses made to a child is MOST likely to reinforce positively the child's appropriate behavior in the dental setting?
A. "You're doing a great job for me today".
B. "I like it when you sit quietly in the chair".
C. "This visit is going really well, don't you think?
D. "Coming to the dentist isn't so bad after all, is it?

11. Which of the following is MOST convenient method for examining an 18 months old child?
A. The child sitting on the dental chair and a parent at the chairside
B. A parent sitting on the dental chair and child on the parent's lap facing forward.
C. The dentist and parent in a knee-to-knee position with the child's head in the dentist's lap.
D. The dentist and parent in a knee-to-knee position with the child's legs in the parent's lap

12. Which of the following generally describes children with defiant behavior?
A. They are usually around 3 years of age or younger
B. They are also referred to as stubborn or spoiled
C. They usually exhibit tremors in voice when speaking
D. They exhibit quiet sobbing with profuse tears

13. During an emergency dental visit, a moderately retarded 4 years old child resists physically and cries excessively. In this instance, the dentist should use which of the following?
A. Physical restraints
B. General anesthesia
C. The hand over mouth exercise
D. Voice control

14. Child abuse/neglect most commonly involves children in which age group?
A. Birth to age three years
B. Four to six years
C. Seven to nine years
D. All age groups are equally affected

15. The basic fear of a child below 2 years on his first dental visit is related to:
A. Anxiety from being separated from parents
B. Fear of infection
C. Fear of bur sound
D. Fear of white apron worn by dentist and nurses

16. A child patient demonstrating resistance in the dental office is usually manifesting:
A. Anxiety
B. Anger
C. Inborn fear
D. Immaturity

17. Extinguishing of fears on successive dental visit, is an example of:
A. Modelling
B. Reinforcement
C. Association
D. Desensitization

Answers

1.D. In general, appointments should not be scheduled to last for more than 20 minutes for two years old or 30 to 45 minutes for a child above 5 years of age (The first appointment may be even shorter).

2.A. Bribery rarely incurs any good result. The child will simply keep on behaving badly in order to get more bribes and concessions.

3.D. Introjection is the attempt by the child to take an undesirable object into the oral cavity.

4.D. Projection is the rejection by the child to an undesirable object into the oral cavity.

5.C. As a child grows his/her behavior pattern is governed by his/her inherited physical, mental and environmental influences. Which is usually evident from the condition of anterior teeth.

6.D. The dentist should praise the child's good behavior and try to proceed quickly and efficiently. Appropriate behavior management techniques are employed whenever necessary.

7.A. One of the most important rewards for the child is approval by pedodontist praise of the behavior and good conduct of the child. Gift be given after the work of the day is over.

8.D. Behavioral management in a child can be done by positive approach, team attitude, Organization, truthfulness, tolerance and flexibility.

9.C. Highly anxious parents affect their child's behavior negatively, especially if the child is under 4 years of age This might be anticipated because of parent-child symbiosis that begins in infancy and gradually diminishes with advancement of age.

10.B. The dental surgeon must be aware of the important part played by his appearance, facial expressions, his attire, movements and above all the use of voice.

11.B. At 18 months of age, child shows an intensified closeness with his parents, experiencing real reparation anxiety if they leave the house for a few hours.

12.B. Defiant behavior is mostly observed in children from ages 6 to 10 years. They become highly cooperative once their confidence is gained by the pedodontist and his auxiliaries.

13.A. Physical restraint is used to protect the patient and / or dental staff from injury and reduce untoward movement while providing dental care.

14.A. Child abuse and neglect include various experiences of a child, which are threatening or harmful. These are always the result of improper conduct and responsibility of a caretaker or parents.

15.A. During the second year the child become involved in a new stage of personality growth, the development of a sense of autonomy.

16.A. Anxiety may be defined as apprehension or source which is unknown. Anxiety is considered a normal and a healthy reaction towards a perceived threat.

17.D. Desensitization technique has been found to be effective in managing phobias including fear of rejection, physical injury, infections, etc.

8

Ectopic Eruption

1. **Ectopic or delayed eruption in the anterior segment of the arch may be due to:**
   A. Presence of supernumerary teeth
   B. Unfavorable sequence of eruption
   C. Discrepancy between size of teeth and size of arch
   D. All of the above

2. **Ectopic eruption is:**
   A. Eruption of tooth before its eruption time
   B. Eruption of tooth at abnormal place
   C. Delayed eruption of a tooth
   D. Eruption of an extra tooth

3. **Common cause of ectopic eruption is:**
   A. Arch length deficiency
   B. Supernumerary tooth
   C. Hereditary
   D. Endocrinal disorders

4. **Which maybe the cause of ectopic eruption of the first permanent molar?**
   A. Smaller maxilla
   B. Abnormal mesial angulation of eruption of the maxillary first permanent molar
   C. Delayed calcification of some affected permanent molars
   D. All of the above

Answers

1.D. Eruption of a tooth at an abnormal place is called as ectopic eruption.

2.B. The exact reasons for an abnormally positioned tooth bud are difficult to explain. It maybe due to crowding, hereditary developmental abnormality or due to an injury that malpositions the tooth during the formative years.

3.A. It is a good clue to sacrifice few teeth, if a harmonious relationship between tooth material and basal bone is to be developed and maintained. It may also indicate possible institution of a planned program or guided extraction.

4.D. Ectopic eruption usually has a significant familial tendency and multifactorial mode of inheritance.

9

Cleft Lip and Cleft Palate and their Management

1. The most common orofacial deformity that produces malocclusion is:

A. Cleft palate
B. Pierre-Robin syndrome
C. Cleidocranial dysostosis
D. Osteogenesis imperfecta

2. The deformity of cleft palate occurs during which trimester of pregnancy:

A. Third
B. Second
C. First
D. Any of the above

3. Patients having cleft lip and palate are generally associated with:

A. Respiratory tract infection and malocclusion
B. Airway obstruction
C. Middle ear infection
D. All of the above

4. What is the etiology of the effect of cleft lip and cleft palate?

A. Gene mutation and chromosomal aberrations
B. Hereditary
C. Parental age
D. All of the above

5. What is the rule of "Tens" for cleft lip surgery?

A. 10 weeks of age, 10 pounds of body weight and 10 gm% of Hb
B. 10 month of age, 10 kg of body weight and 10 gm% of Hb
C. 10 years of age, 10 kg of body weight and 10 gm% of Hb
D. None of the above

6. Which of the following is a surgical procedure to treat the cleft lip?

A. Cald-Well-Luc operation
B. Franklin-Inkwell procedure
C. Mirault's procedure
D. None of the above

7. Closure of cleft palate should be done between:

A. 0 to 1 year of age
B. 2 to 4 years of age
C. 1 year to 2 years of age
D. 3 to 5 years of age

Answers

1.A. Cleft lip and palate is a very common congenital deformity of orofacial structures. These defects are present in various clinical forms.

2.C. Clefts of primary palate take place at fifth to eighth week of intrauterine life, while clefts of secondary palate occur between ninth to eleventh weeks of intrauterine life.

3.D. Cleft lip and palate may also result in feeding problem due to malformed teeth and malocclusion, speech problems and dental problems (malformed teeth, malocclusion and partial anodontia).

4.D. Like other congenital deformities, cleft lip and cleft palate are due to multifactorial basis.

5.A. A general rule of "Tens" (10 weeks of age , 10 pounds of body weight and atleast 10 gm percent hemoglobin) is frequently used in determining optimum timing for cleft lip surgery.

6.C. Most of the surgeons prefer to wait for 2 to 3 months before the surgery. They believe that increased size of the lip structure is easier to work with and gives better final results.

7.C. The main purpose of palate closure by the age of 2 years is to facilitate the development of normal speech which correlates with age.

10

Nutrition and Dental Health Care

1. **Which of the following may cause defective formation of teeth?**
   A. Vit. B deficiency
   B. Vit E. deficiency
   C. Maternal or neonatal vitamin A deficiency
   D. None of the above

2. **Biochemical composition and function of salivary glands can be affected by:**
   A. Maternal and neonatal protein deficiency
   B. Maternal and neonatal vitamin deficiency
   C. Maternal and neonatal fat deficiency
   D. None of the above

3. **Which is the most cariogenic?**
   A. Glucose
   B. Fructose
   C. Sucrose
   D. Starch

4. **Fats have an anticariogenic effect because:**
   A. Fermentable substrate is prevented from its entry into the plaque by covering the plaque with a layer of fat
   B. Fat layer on the tooth surface prevents food retention
   C. Increase in fat in diet decreases the carbohydrate content of diet
   D. All of the above are correct

5. **Due to the deficiency of protein in diet in children, which of the following is observed?**
   A. Smaller teeth size
   B. More caries prone teeth
   C. Crowded and rotated teeth
   D. All of the above

6. Which of the following is not a carcinogenic sweetener?
A. Fructose
B. Invert sugar
C. Xylitol
D. Cyclamate

7. Deficiency of vit. A in children can cause:
A. Hyperplasia and hyperkeratosis of gingival tissues
B. Hypoplastic and chalky-white incisors
C. Atrophy of odontoblasts
D. All of the above

8. Vitamin 'D' deficiency causes:
A. Hypocalcification and hypoplasia of enamel and dentin
B. Appearance of calciotraumatic line
C. Both of the above
D. None of the above

9. Vitamin 'E' deficiency causes:
A. Chalky-white teeth
B. Disarrangement of ameloblasts
C. Both of the above
D. None

10. Vitamin 'C' deficiency causes:
A. Marginal gingival enlargement
B. Gingiva becomes hemorrhagic
C. Poor resistance to infection
D. All of the above

11. Deficiency of 'Ca' and 'P' can cause:
A. Increased dental caries
B. Altered calcification
C. Defective bone formation
D. All of the above

Answers

1.C. Maternal or neonatal vitamin A deficiency may cause defective formation of teeth. Maternal and neonatal protein deficiency affects the biochemical composition and function of salivary glands.

2.A. Saliva helps in remineralization and has some immunosuppressive action. So alteration in salivary function due to early protein deficiency may cause increase in caries susceptibility.

3.C. Sugar (sucrose) is cheap, easily purified and high in calories. An ideal sugar substitute must have the physical properties like sugar.

4.D. Fat have an anticariogenic effect. Highly concentrated fatty acids inhibit the growth of cariogenic bacteria.

5.D. Protein deficiency also results in late third molar eruption or no eruption at all, breakdown of cancellous bone and retarded cementum deposition.

6.D. Cyclamate is an organic sweetener. It is about 30 times sweeter than sucrose currently banned in the USA as a possible carcinogen.

7.D. Enamel hypoplasia, if combined with local cariogenic factors, results in rampant caries of the deciduous anterior teeth.

8.C. Hypoplastic lesions are more prominent in the incisors, canines and in the first permanent molars.

9.C. Sources of vitamin E are meat, butter, milk, fish liver oil, green leaves, wheat germ oil, cotton seed oil, peanut oil, etc.

10.D. Vitamin C deficiency causes hemorrhage, collagen degeneration and edema of the gingival connective tissue. Deficiency of Vitamin C alone does not produce gingivitis, local irritation is necessary to initiate the inflammatory reaction.

11.D. Severe dietary deficiency of calcium or Vitamin D, Vitamin D resistant rickets or intake of tetracycline will cause enamel hypoplasia, hypocalcification and pigmentation.

11

Toothbrushing Methods for Children

1. **Which method of brushing provides good stimulation to the gingiva?**
   - **A.** Fones method
   - **B.** Scrub method
   - **C.** Bass method
   - **D.** Press role method
2. **Which of the following brushing methods is good for children in mixed dentition stage?**
   - **A.** Fones method
   - **B.** Scrub method
   - **C.** Bass method
   - **D.** Rolling stroke or press role method
3. **Which of the following represents the MOST effective way of encouraging a child to floss regularly?**
   - **A.** Presenting a message that concerns the potential loss of teeth if the patient does not floss
   - **B.** Arranging for the child to earn privileges for flossing
   - **C.** Repeating periodically the message on the value of flossing
   - **D.** Providing written material that explains the mechanism of flossing

Answers

1.A. Fones method is easy to learn for the children. Good stimulation is provided to the gingiva.

2.D. Rolling stroke or Press role method is good for general cleaning of teeth and stimulation of gingiva.

3.B. The various individual factors which determine the choice of dental floss are the tightness of tooth contacts the roughness of tooth surfaces and the patient's manual dextrin.

12

Normal Periodontium and Periodontal Diseases in Children

1. **Which of the following is same as dental plaque?**
   A. Pellicle
   B. Materia alba
   C. Debris
   D. None of the above
2. **What causes the green stains frequently seen on children's teeth?**
   A. Chromogenic bacteria
   B. Materia alba
   C. Enamel defects
   D. Dentin defects
3. **What is the common cause of draining fistulas in gingival tissue of children?**
   A. Chronic periapical abscess
   B. Acute periodontal abscess
   C. Acute periapical abscess
   D. Periapical cysts
4. **Normal color of gingiva is:**
   A. Red B. Bluish-red
   C. Dark pink D. Pale-pink
5. **Which of the following statements is correct about the Down's syndrome?**
   A. In Down's syndrome, children are highly caries susceptible
   B. The children have lower rate of periodontal disease
   C. Children suffer from high caries and low periodontal disease
   D. Children suffer from high periodontal diseases

6. **Herpetic gingivostomatitis is caused by:**
   A. Herpes zoster virus
   B. Herpes simplex virus
   C. Both of the above
   D. None of the above

7. **Which of the following is correct about the juvenile periodontitis?**
   A. Its onset is during circum pubertal period
   B. It shows familial tendency
   C. It shows rapid loss of bone destruction
   D. All of the above

8. **Hypophosphatasia:**
   A. Is a rare hereditary condition
   B. Results in premature loss of the deciduous teeth
   C. Results in minimal gingival inflammation associated with loss of tooth
   D. All of the above are correct

9. **Papillon-Lefevre syndrome is characterized by:**
   A. Destruction of supporting tissues of the deciduous teeth only
   B. Destruction of supporting tissues of the permanent teeth only
   C. Destruction of supporting tissues of the deciduous and permanent teeth and hyperkeratosis of soles and palms
   D. None of the above

10. **Causative organism of "cellulitis" is:**
    A. Staphylococci B. Streptococci
    C. *E. Coli* D. Actinomycosis

11. **Which of the following represents the most common form of gingival periodontal disease in school-aged children?**
    A. Juvenile periodontitis
    B. Localized acute gingivitis
    C. Primary herpetic gingivostomatitis
    D. Necrotizing ulcerative gingivitis

Answers

1.D. Pellicle is deposited on tooth soon after its eruption in oral cavity. The transition from pellicle to dental plaque is extremely rapid. At the gingival margins, the collection of debris consists of bacteria and epithelial cells. It is called material alba, which is usually of dirty white color.

2.A. In children the most common is green stain. It is observed on the labial surface of incisors and canines in both the maxillary and mandibular teeth. It is more common in boys than in girls.

3.A. Chromic periapical abscess drain in the path of least resistance. Gingival tissues offer the path of least resistance.

4.D. The gingiva is normally firm, pale-pink in color. The color is related to the complexion of the face, thickness of the tissue and degree of keratinization.

5.D. Advanced periodontal disease with deep periodontal pockets has been associated with Down's syndrome. There is horizontal type alveolar bone loss of 5 mm or more.

6.B. The children are usually affected at the age of 1 and 3 years. The gingiva displays a fiery-red inflammation, a loss of distinction between the attached gingiva and the alveolar mucosa.

7.C. Juvenile periodontitis is characterized by migration and loosening of the teeth in the presence or absence of either secondary epithelial proliferation and pocket formation or secondary gingival disease.

8.D. Tooth loss in hypophosphatasia is due to insufficient periodontal ligament attachment because of the cemental defect.

9.C. Gingival swelling precedes destruction of the periodontium. Bony destruction is severe along with complete loss of the alveolar process.

10.B. Cellulitis is a diffuse inflammation of the soft tissues that may be caused by a pulpless deciduous or permanent tooth. Streptococci are common causative organisms in cases of cellulitis and are particularly potent producers of hyaluronidase.

11.B. About 60% of the teenagers have gingival bleeding on probing. Gingivitis in children is largely reversible.

13

Dental Caries

1. **Which of the following items is probably the least cariogenic:**
   A. Cookie
   B. Soft drink
   C. Ice cream
   D. Toffee

2. **In nursing bottle rampant caries, usually teeth involved are:**
   A. All primary teeth
   B. Primary maxillary incisors and primary first molar
   C. Primary mandibular incisor and primary first molar
   D. Only primary mandibular incisors

3. **Acidogenic theory was given by:**
   A. W D Miller
   B. G V Black
   C. Schatz
   D. Anderson

4. **Proteolysis-chelation theory was given by:**
   A. W D Miller
   B. G Black
   C. Schatz
   D. Anderson

5. **Which of the following elements has cariogenic property?**
   A. Sodium
   B. Magnesium
   C. Lithium
   D. Molybdenum

6. **Which of the following elements is not cariostatic?**
   A. Molybdenum
   B. Vanadium
   C. Cadmium
   D. Strontium

7. **Pellicle consists mainly of:**
   A. Fat
   B. Protein
   C. Glycoproteins
   D. All of the above

8. **The function of the pellicle is:**
   A. To protect the enamel
   B. To reduce the friction between the teeth
   C. Possibly to provide a matrix for remineralization
   D. All of the above

9. **In deciduous dentition, the caries follows a specific pattern which is:**
   A. Mandibular molars, maxillary molars and maxillary anterior teeth
   B. Maxillary anterior, maxillary molars and mandibular molars
   C. Mandibular anterior, maxillary molars and mandibular molars
   D. Maxillary molar, mandibular anteriors and maxillary anterior teeth

10. **The causative organism for initiation of enamel caries is:**
   A. Streptococci
   B. Staphylococci
   C. *A. viscosus*
   D. Lactobacilli

11. **The causative organism of root caries is:**
   A. Streptococci
   B. Staphylococci
   C. Lactobacilli
   D. *A. viscosus*

12. **Which organism is important in progression of dentinal caries?**
   A. Streptococci
   B. Staphylococci
   C. Lactobacilli
   D. *E. Coli*

13. **Nursing bottle caries is an example of:**
   A. Acute dental caries
   B. Smooth surface caries
   C. Pit and fissure caries
   D. Chronic dental caries

14. **What is the characteristic feature of rampant caries?**
   A. It involves caries immune surfaces
   B. Proximal surfaces of anterior lower incisors are also involved
   C. Development of cervical caries also takes place
   D. All of the above are correct

15. **Arrested caries:**
   A. Occurs only in deciduous teeth
   B. Occurs only in permanent teeth
   C. Occurs in both deciduous and permanent teeth
   D. Is very rapidly growing caries

16. **Arrested caries:**
    A. Occurs in both deciduous and permanent dentition
    B. Occurs on occlusal and proximal surfaces
    C. Does not retain food
    D. All of the above are correct

17. **Nursing bottle caries can also be called as:**
    A. Nursing bottle syndrome
    B. Milk bottle syndrome
    C. Early childhood caries
    D. All of the above

18. **Etiological risk factor of nursing bottle caries is:**
    A. Feeding beyond the weaning age i.e. beyond 12 to 15 months
    B. Immuno-compromised children
    C. Children with sleep disorder
    D. All of the above

19. **Besides milk, other food product/s responsible for nursing caries is/are:**
    A. Fruit juice
    B. Honey
    C. Sweetened beverages
    D. All of the above

20. **Which of the following teeth are usually affected by nursing bottle caries?**
    A. Maxillary incisors B. Mandibular molars
    C. Mandibular incisors D. Maxillary molars

Answers

1.B. Cookie, toffee and ice cream are not recommended as a dessert or in between meals for caries susceptible patients.

2.B. Nursing bottle caries is easily recognizable and a distinct pattern of dental decay affecting specific teeth to a greater or lesser extent.

3.A. Acidogenic theory was given by WD Miller in 1882.

4.C. Reduced incidence of dental caries due to fluoridation can be explained by proteolysis chelation theory.

5.B. The elements such as selenium, magnesium and cadmium are considered to be cariogenic.

6.C. The elements molybdenum, vanadium and strontium are considered to be cariostatic.

7.C. Pellicle consists mainly of glycoproteins, different carbohydrates and immunoglobulins.

8.D. The pellicle is formed primarily from the selective precipitation of various components of saliva to apatite surface.

9.A. The second deciduous molars in both the mandibular and maxillary arches are more susceptible to dental caries because the occlusal surface of the teeth has deeper less completely coalesced pits and fissures.

10.A. The causative organisms for initiation of enamel caries are streptococci. They secrete enzyme glucoxyltransferase which enhances the polymerization of the extracellular matrix and makes mutans streptococci to form much tenaciously adherent colonies.

11.D. *Actinomycosis viscosus* is the causative organism of root caries.

12.C. Lactobacilli are important in the progression of dentinal caries because of its acidogenic potential.

13.A. Acute dental type of caries follows a rapid clinical course and results in early pulp involvement.

14.D. Rampant caries is a suddenly appearing, widespread, rapidly burrowing type of caries, resulting in early involvement of the pulp and affecting those teeth usually regarded as immune to ordinary decay.

15.C. When the carious process after initiation and actual disintegration of tooth surface does not proceed further and is arrested because the area becomes self-cleansing, it is called arrested caries.

16.D. This type of caries is relatively uncommon and does not have any tendency for further progression, as it becomes static or stationary.

17.D. Other names of nursing bottle caries are baby bottle tooth decay and nursing caries.

18.D. Other etiological risk factors include feeding at night, high socioeconomic status, low socioeconomic status, single parent and a strong temperamental child.

19.D. Mother's milk remains the ideal food for a child despite the cariogenic potential. It is sweeter as compared to bovine milk because of its higher lactose content.

20.A. It involves the lingual, mesial, distal and labial surfaces of maxillary primary incisors, especially burrowing the cervical region of the teeth and the occlusal, buccal lingual surfaces of maxillary and mandibular molars, the mandibular incisors are usually spared.

14

Caries Activity Tests

1. **Dental caries activity test is/are:**
   A. Snyder's test
   B. Oricult test
   C. Swab test
   D. All of the above

2. **Lactobacillus seems to be mainly involved with the:**
   A. Initiation of dental caries
   B. Progression of carious lesion
   C. Both of the above
   D. None of the above

3. **Optimum pH for growth of Lactobacilli is:**
   A. 4.0
   B. 5.0
   C. 6.0
   D. 7.0

4. **Which caries activity test is ideal for patient education?**
   A. Lactobacilli count
   B. Snyder's test
   C. Alban's test
   D. All of the above

Answers

1.D. Caries activity is defined as "the sum of new carious lesion and enlargement of existing cavities during a certain time period".

2.B. Lactobacillus are acidogenic and acidouric. They are often found in the deeper parts of a caries lesion. The Lactobacillus count can be used both for estimation of caries risk and for control of dietary changes.

3.A. Although Lactobacillus colony count test is quick and easy, the results are not available for several days. Also counting colonies is a tedious process and complex equipment and personnel are required.

4.C. Alban's test is good for indicating caries inactivity. Alban's test is very simple, can be performed in the clinic of the private practitioner and is ideal for patient education.

15

Prevention of Dental Caries and Periodontal Diseases in Children

1. **For an effective plaque removal from teeth of caries susceptible infant:**
   - A. Teeth should be brushed twice daily by the parent
   - B. Teeth should be brushed thoroughly once daily by the parent preferably in the morning
   - C. Teeth should be brushed thoroughly once a day only by the infant preferably in the morning
   - D. None of the above
2. **Mother's milk is ideal food for a child because:**
   - A. It is the perfect food at the perfect temperature
   - B. It provides a natural transfer of immunoglobulins
   - C. Development of orofacial structures occurs due to continuous sucking
   - D. All of the above
3. **Which of the following is used in prevention of dental caries?**
   - A. Magnesium chloride
   - B. Sodium chloride
   - C. Zinc chloride
   - D. None of the above
4. **Which vitamin is used in prevention of dental caries?**
   - A. Vitamin A B. Vitamin D
   - C. Vitamin K D. Vitamin E
5. **The most common method of removing plaque form the oral cavity is:**
   - A. Chlorhexidine B. Tooth brushing
   - C. Alexidine D. All of the above

6. The most effective method to prevent the formation of plaque:

A. Tooth brushing
B. Flossing
C. Chlorhexidine
D. All of the above

7. Which of the following is not a disclosing agent?

A. Gention violet
B. Erythrocin
C. Tetracycline
D. Fluorescein

8. Which of the following is a plaque attachment interference agent?

A. Kanamycin sulfate
B. Urea peroxide
C. Chlorhexidine
D. Sodium polyvinyl phosphoric acid

9. Which of the following antibiotics is used as a chemical plaque control agent?

A. Pencillin
B. Tetracycline
C. Vancomycin HCl
D. All of the above

10. Which of the following enzymes is used as a chemical plaque controlling agent?

A. Mucinases
B. Pancreatin
C. Proteases
D. All of the above

11. Plaque accumulation can be prevented by:

A. Pit and fissure sealant
B. Fissure eradication
C. Tooth surface conditioning
D. All of the above

12. Caries can be controlled by:

A. Increasing tooth surface resistance
B. Improving morphology of tooth
C. Increasing detersive roughage in diet
D. All of the above

13. Caries can be controlled and prevented:

A. If salivary flow is increased
B. If buffering ability of saliva is increased
C. If stickiness of saliva is reduced
D. All of the above

14. Chlorhexidine gluconate is very effective in reducing plaque in which minimum concentration:

A. 0.1 % **B.** 0.2 %
C. 0.3 % **D.** 0.4 %

15. Anticalculus dentifrices contain:

A. Tetra sodium pyrophosphate (3.4%)
B. Disodium dihydrogen pyrophosphate (1.37%)
C. $ZnCl_2$
D. All of the above

16. In a preschool child, common cause of acute generalized gingival inflammation is:

A. Pyogenic granuloma
B. Vitamin deficiency
C. Scurvy
D. Acute herpetic gingivostomatitis

Answers

1.A. Parents should brush the teeth of small children who have not yet learnt proper handling of the toothbrushes or not gained coordination.

2.D. A bond of love and affection is formed between the infant and the mother which provides the child with a much needed security and warmth.

3.C. Howe reported that the application of ammonical silver nitrate, zinc chloride and potassium ferrocyanide solutions to the tooth surface may reduce the incidence of dental caries. These chemicals diffuse into the enamel and dentin and complexes are formed with proteins of enamel and dentin which are less soluble in acids.

4.C. Vitamin K act by interfering with the carbohydrate degradation through enzymatic alterations.

5.B. Plaque can be controlled by the patient himself by the use of toothbrush, flossing and interdental cleasnsing oral irrigation and the use of fluoride in the form of mouthwash, toothpaste, mouthrinse and gels.

6.C. Daily rinses twice a day with a 10 ml of 0.2 percent aqueous solution almost completely inhibit the development of dental plaque, calculus, gingivitis.

7.C. Disclosing agents is a chemical preparation containing dye or other coloring agent. It is used to locate and identity bacterial plaque deposits on teeth, tongue and gingiva.

8.D. Perfluoroalkyl is also plaque attachment interference agent.

9.C. Penicillin, Vancomycin and tetracyclin are the three antibiotics which have been studied for their use against plaque and gingivitis, but it is inappropriate for routine use in plaque control.

10.D. Mucinases, pancreatin, fungal enzymes and proteases are used as a chemical plaque controlling agent.

11.D. Prevention for plaque accumulation rendered by professional services by changing the tooth morphology include pit and fissure sealants, prophylactic odontomy, fissure eradication and tooth surface conditioning by LASER.

12. D. Caries can be controlled by decreased bacterial growth, decreased plaque formation, decreased bacterial enzyme activity of decreased carbohydrate-bacterial activity .

13.D. Caries can also be controlled and prevented by increasing the nonsticky and watery contents of saliva. Saliva also helps to increase remineralization of demineralized tooth surface.

14.B. Daily rinses twice a day with a 10 mL of 0.2 percent aqueous solution almost completely inhibit the development of dental plaque ,calculus, gingivitis.

15.D. Anticalculus dentifrices contain calculus controlling agents like tetrasodium pyrophosphate (3.4%), disodium dihydrogen pyrophosphate (1.37%) and zinc chloride(2%).

16.D. Acute herpetic gingivostomatitis is inflammatory condition caused by the herpes simplex virus. The children are usually affected at the age of 1and 3 years.

16

Pathology of Soft Oral Tissues and Jaws

1. Mucocele is commonly found in:
A. Upper lip B. Lower lip
C. Floor of the mouth D. Tongue

2. Fibrous dysplasia is a:
A. Neoplastic lesion
B. Non-neoplastic lesion
C. Inflammatory lesion
D. Traumatic lesion

3. Albright's syndrome is a:
A. Hereditary condition
B. Severe form of monostotic fibrous dysplasia
C. Severe form of polystotic fibrous dysplasia
D. Trisomy of 12th chromosome

4. Monostotic fibrous dysplasia more frequently involves the:
A. Maxilla
B. Mandible
C. Both jaws are equally involved
D. Can not predict

5. Cementifying fibroma originates from:
A. Rest cell of Malassez
B. Degeneration of the enamel organ
C. Periodontal ligament
D. Accumulation of water between reduced enamel epithelium and enamel organ

6. Central giant cell granuloma:
A. Commonly occurs in the 3rd decade of life
B. Is more common in females
C. Is more common in mandible
D. All of the above

7. Ameloblastoma is more common in:
A. Maxilla
B. Mandible
C. Equal in both the jaws
D. Cannot predict

8. Ameloblastoma is commonly found in:
A. Molar ramus region
B. Anterior region of mandible
C. Anterior region of maxilla
D. Canine region of mandible

9. Which of these is not a true cyst?
A. Primordial cyst
B. Residual cyst
C. Aneurysmal bone cyst
D. Globulomaxillary cyst

10. Which of the following is not an odontogenic cyst?
A. Residual cyst
B. Incisive canal cyst
C. Dentigerous cyst
D. Lateral periodontal cyst

11. For a lesion of the size of 2 mm, the biopsy performed usually is:
A. Needle biopsy
B. Incisional biopsy
C. Fine needle aspiration cytology
D. Excisional biopsy

12. For a salivary gland neoplasm or a lymph node, the biopsy usually performed is:
A. Fine needle aspiration cytology
B. Incisional biopsy
C. Excisional biopsy
D. Needle biopsy

Answers

1.B. Mucocele or mucous retention cyst is a salivary gland lesion of traumatic origin.

2.B. Fibrous dysplasia is a non-neoplastic developmental lesion of bone.

3.C. Albright's syndrome is a severe form of polyostotic fibrous dysplasia associated with café an lait macules on the skin, Cushing's syndrome, hyperthyroidism, hyperparathy – roidism, diabetes mellitus and precocious puberty .

4.A. Monostotic fibrous dysplasia is seen with nearly equal frequency in males and females .

5.C. Ossifying and cementifying fibroma is a benign fibro-osseous neoplasm originating form periodontal ligament. It can occur at any age, but is more common in teenagers.

6.D. Giant cell granuloma is a common reactive lesion of the bone. Usually, it occurs in the anterior portion of jaw.

7.B. Ameloblastoma usually occurs in second to fourth decade of life with 80 percent of cases occuring in the mandible and out of these, over 70 percent in the molar ramus region.

8.A. Ameloblastoma is usually a benign odontogenic locally invasive neoplasm of enamel forming cells and is persistent and aggressive in nature.

9.C. Primordial cyst arises due to degeneration of the enamel organ. In this, a cyst is formed instead of a tooth.

10.B. Incisive canal cyst is the most common fissural cyst .It is derived form vestigial elements of the embryologic nasopalatine duct located in the incisive canal .

11.D. Excisional biopsy is the biopsy of a tissue removed by surgical cutting .This is preferred if the size of the lesion is small enough such that it may be removed along with a margin of normal tissue for microscopic study.

12.A. FNAC is the biopsy in which tissue is obtained by puncture of a tumor, the tissue within the lumen of the needle being detached by rotation and the needle withdrawn.

17

Development of Occlusion

1. **The "Ugly Duckling Stage" of dentition in a child is corrected by the eruption of which tooth?**
   A. Canine
   B. 1st premolar
   C. Lateral incisor
   D. Central incisor

2. **The average Leeway space in an individual is:**
   A. 0.9 mm in maxilla and 1.7 mm in mandible
   B. 0.9 mm in mandible and 1.7 mm in maxilla
   C. 0.7 mm in mandible and 1.9 mm in maxilla
   D. 1.7 mm in maxilla and 1.9 mm in mandible

3. **Name of the space between the lateral incisor and the canine in maxillary deciduous teeth is:**
   A. Leeway space
   B. Primate space
   C. Bolton space
   D. Freeway space

4. **Toothbuds generally initiated after birth are:**
   A. Variable
   B. All permanent and some primary teeth
   C. Entire permanent dentition
   D. First and second premolars and second and third molar only

5. **If the distal surface of the maxillary second molar is distal to the mandibular 2nd primary molar, it depicts:**
   A. Distal step relationship
   B. Mesial step relationship
   C. Straight terminal plane relationship
   D. None of the above

6. **With the eruption of which teeth do maxillary anterior diastemas normally close:**
   A. Canines
   B. First molars
   C. Third molars
   D. Premolars

7. **How much incisor liability is found in maxillary arch?**
   A. 5 mm
   B. 6 mm
   C. 7 mm
   D. 8 mm

8. **In mandibular teeth, incisor liability is:**
   A. 4 mm
   B. 5 mm
   C. 6 mm
   D. 7 mm

9. **At the age of 6 to 7 years in the primary dentition, the inter dental spacing in maxilla usually ranges:**
   A. Between 0 and 10 mm
   B. Between 0 and 5 mm
   C. Between 0 and 15 mm
   D. Between 0 and 20 mm

10. **Incisor crowding may be assessed by:**
    A. Interdental spacing
    B. Intercanine arch width
    C. Labiolingual incisor position
    D. All of the above

11. **Pigeon profile of face is found in the:**
    A. Class I type 3 malocclusion
    B. Class II div 1 malocclusion
    C. Class II div 2 malocclusion
    D. Class III malocclusion

12. **Class III malocclusion is best treated in:**
    A. Deciduous and mixed dentition period
    B. Mixed and permanent dentition period
    C. Early permanent dentition period
    D. Can be treated at any age

13. **Primate spaces are present:**
    A. Mesial to primary canine in maxilla and distal to primary canine in mandible
    B. Mesial to primary canine in both arches
    C. Distal to primary canine in maxilla and mesial to primary canine in mandible
    D. Distal to primary canine in both the arches

14. The most common space in the primary dentition is:

A. Physiological space **B.** Developmental space
C. Primate space **D.** None

15. Terminal plane is:

A. Relation between distal surfaces of upper and lower second primary molar
B. Relation between mesial surfaces of upper and lower second primary molar
C. Relation between distal surfaces of upper and lower first primary molar
D. Relation between mesial surfaces of upper and lower first primary molar

16. Molar relation in primary dentition is called as mesial step when:

A. Distal surface of upper and lower second primary molar are in straight line
B. Distal surface of lower second molar is distal to that of upper
C. Distal surface of lower second molar is mesial to that of upper
D. Distal surface of upper second molar is mesial to that of lower

17. Arch width increases up to:

A. 6 years of age
B. 12 years of age
C. 14 years of age
D. 18 years of age

18. A flush terminal plane relationship in primary dentition usually results in:

A. Class III molar relation in permanent dentition
B. Class II molar relationship in permanent dentition
C. Class I molar relationship in permanent dentition
D. Cannot be predicted

19. Mesial step relationship in primary dentition results into:

A. Class I molar relationship in permanent dentition
B. Class II molar relationship in permanent
C. Class III molar relationship in permanent dentition
D. Cannot be predicted dentition

20. Distal step relationship in primary dentition results into:
- **A.** Class I molar relationship in permanent dentition
- **B.** Class II molar relationship in permanent dentition
- **C.** Class III molar relation
- **D.** Cannot be predicted

21. Which one of the following is a self-correcting condition?
- **A.** Ugly-duckling stage
- **B.** Primate space
- **C.** Physiologic space
- **D.** All of the above

22. In the case of bimaxillary protrusion, interincisal angle is:
- **A.** Increased
- **B.** Decreased
- **C.** Normal
- **D.** None of the above

Answers

1.A. In ugly duckling stage, which is a self- correcting condition, permanent central incisors have strong distal inclination. It occurs at the age of around 8 to 9 years.

2.B. The sum total of mesiodistal dimension of CDE is always greater than 345. Excess space, referred to as leeway space, is important for allowing adjustment of first molar relationship.

3.B. The most common spaces in the deciduous dentition are the spaces mesial to deciduous canine in the maxilla and distal to deciduous canine in the mandible. These spaces are called the primate spaces and are characteristic of deciduous dentition.

4.D. If a child loses his primary molars at or before 5 years of age, the eruption of premolars will be delayed.

5.B. Mesial step of deciduous dentition results in direct eruption of permanent first molars into Class I occlusion.

6.A. The transitional malalignment during the exchange period of the upper incisors is called "The ugly duckling stage". This is corrected when the canines erupt and the pressure is transferred from the roots to the crowns of the incisors.

7.C. The sum total of mesiodistal dimensions of 4 permanent incisors is more than that of 4 deciduous incisors by about 7 mm in maxilla and 5 mm in mandible .

8.B. Spacing allows relatively larger permanent incisors to be accomodated in the arch.

9.A. The physiological spaces that exist in the primary dentition are important factors in allowing the relatively large permanent incisors to be accomodated in the arch.

10.D. The intercanine width increases remarkably at the time of eruption of the maxillary central incisors and the mandibular lateral incisors.

11.B. Class II div 1 malocclusion is disto-occlusion in which the maxillary central incisors are typically in extreme labioversion .

12.A. In Class III malocclusion, the mandibular first permanent molar exists in mesio-occlusion by almost a full premolar width.

13.A. Primate spaces are characteristic of deciduous dentition .The other spaces in deciduous dentition are called developmental spaces.

14.C. Primate space of maxillary arch is also known as Baum's space.

15.A. The mesiodistal relation of the distal surface of the upper and lower second primary molar is called the terminal plane when the primary teeth contact in centric occlusion.

16.C. Molar relation in primary dentition is called as distal step when the distal surface of the lower molar is more distal to that of upper.

17.A. Arch width in anterior region after 6 years of age does not increase .

18.C. In flush terminal plane, distal surfaces of upper and lower second deciduous molars are flushed in straight line .

19.A. Mesial step of deciduous dentition results in direct eruption of permanent first molars into Class I occlusion.

20.B. An exaggerated mesial step leads to Class III malocclusion, while distal step terminal plane always leads to Class II occlusion.

21.D. The transitional malalignment during the exchange period of the upper incisors is called "The Ugly Duckling Stage". This is corrected later when the canines erupt and the pressure is transferred from the roots to the crowns of the incisors .

22.B. In bimaxillary protrusion , molar relations are normal but both the jaws are placed anteriorly.

18

Classification of Malocclusion

1. **In a Class I malocclusion, the mesiobuccal cusp of the maxillary first permanent molar will be in:**
   A. Relation to the embrasure between the first and second premolars
   B. Relation to embrasure between mandibular first and second molar
   C. Relation to embrasure between mandibular second premolar and first molar
   D. Correct mesiodistal relation to the mesiobuccal groove of the mandibular first permanent molar

2. **Among the clearly established local causes, the most common cause of malocclusion is:**
   A. Tongue thrusting
   B. Thumb sucking
   C. Premature loss of deciduous teeth
   D. Prolonged retention of deciduous teeth

3. **The most common local cause of malocclusion is:**
   A. Congenital absence of third molars
   B. Late eruption of permanent teeth
   C. Presence of supernumerary teeth
   D. Thumb sucking habit

4. **Angle's Class I type malocclusion is characterized by:**
   A. Molar in Class I relation with crowded and rotated incisors
   B. Molar in Class II relation with spacing between incisors
   C. Molar in Class I relation with spacing between incisors
   D. Molar in Class II relation with crowded and rotated incisors

5. **Characteristic feature of Angle's Class II type II malocclusion is:**
   A. Class I molar with spaced upper incisors
   B. Class I molar with spaced lower incisors
   C. Class I molar with spaced upper and lower incisors
   D. None of the above

6. **Characteristic feature of Angle's Class I type III malocclusion is:**
   A. Molar in Class I with anterior crowding
   B. Molar in Class I with anterior cross bite
   C. Molar in Class I with posterior cross bite
   D. Molar in Class I with spacing between incisors

7. **Angle's classification:**
   A. Classifies the group of malocclusion
   B. Informs maxillary and mandibular jaw relationship
   C. Informs maxillary and mandibular pattern of growth
   D. All of the above

8. **Dewey's modification of Angle's classification is:**
   A. Class I is divided into five types and Class III into three types
   B. Class I is divided into three types and Class II into five types
   C. Class I is divided into five types and Class II into three types
   D. Class I is divided into three types and Class III in five types

Answers

1.D. Class I malocclusion is a group of malocclusion with normal anteroposterior relationship of molars.

2.B. Thumb sucking condition results in typical labial flaring of maxillary anterior teeth with lingual collapse of mandibular incisors.

3.D. The presence of thumb sucking habit upto 2½ to 3 years of age is considered norma. Persistence of this habit beyond 3½ years of age can have a damaging influence on the dentoalveolar structures and should be intercepted.

4.A. Class I malocclusion is a group of malocclusion with normal anteroposterior relationship of molars but one or more of the following defects:

- Crowding
- Spacing
- Open bite
- Scissors bite
- Missing teeth.

5.D. There is no modification in Angle's Class II malocclusion .

6.B. Characteristic feature of Angles's Class I type I malocclusion is crowded anterior teeth. Type II-Maxillary incisors in labioversion.

Type III Anterior cross bite

Type IV Posterior cross bite

Type V Mesial migration of molars

7.D. Angle's classification also informs maxillary and mandibular first molar relationship.

8.A. Martin Dewey in 1915 modified and divided Angle's classification, there is no modification in Class II.

19

Cephalometric Techniques: Analysis and Interpretations

1. Cephalometrics is used in orthodontics to:

A. Study growth changes
B. Aid in diagnosis and case analysis
C. Treat malocclusions
D. Both A and B

2. In cephalometric analysis of children with malocclusion, the angle ANB is frequently used. In patients with severe Class II malocclusion, this angle is:

A. Large **B.** Small
C. Normal **D.** Negative

3. Distance between cephalostat and an X-ray tube should be:

A. 3 feet **B.** 4 feet
C. 5 feet **D.** 6 feet

4. In cephalogram, the film size used is:

A. 4 x 8 inch **B.** 6 x 8 inch
C. 8 x 10 inch **D.** 6 x 10 inch

5. In cephalogram, point 'A' is:

A. The most anterior projection of the anterior nasal spine (ANS) of the maxilla in the medial plane
B. The deepest point of the curvature of the anterior maxilla between ANS and the alveolar crest
C. The most posterior point on the outer curve of the mandibular anterior process
D. None of the above

6. In cephalogram, Menton (M) is:
- **A.** The most anterior point on the mid-sagittal mandibular symphysis
- **B.** The most inferior point of the mandibular symphysis
- **C.** A constructed point which is formed by the intersection of the facial and mandibular planes
- **D.** None of the above

7. In cephalogram, the Basion (Ba) is:
- **A.** The most inferio-posterior point on the occipital bone
- **B.** Most superior point of external auditory meatus
- **C.** The intersection of the inferior border of the foramen rotundum
- **D.** None of the above

8. Frankfort-horizontal plane is constructed from:
- **A.** Porion to orbitale
- **B.** Porion to A.N.S.(Anterior nasal spine)
- **C.** From Basion (Ba) to Nasion (N)
- **D.** Point A to Point B

9. Facial plane is constructed through:
- **A.** The Nasion perpendicular to the mandibular plane
- **B.** Perpendicular to occlusal plane
- **C.** Perpendicular to B.N. plane
- **D.** The Nasion perpendicular to the Frankfort horizontal plane

10. Which of the following is correct?
- **A.** Normal value of A.N.B angle is +4°
- **B.** A.N.B. angle is always positive
- **C.** If A.N.B. angle is negative that indicates a Class III skeletal relationship
- **D.** A.N.B. angle is always negative

11. Normal value of the maxillary incisor angulation is:
- **A.** 100° **B.** 101°
- **C.** 102° **D.** 103°

12. Which of the following is not a cephalometric analysis?
- **A.** Tweed's analysis **B.** Steiner's analysis
- **C.** Holdaway's analysis **D.** None of the above

13. Facial angle determines:

A. Location of maxilla in horizontal position
B. Location of the horizontal position of the chin
C. Location of the horizontal position of the maxilla and mandible bone
D. All of the above

14. Cephalometric radiographs are useful for the:

A. Location of the origin of malocclusion
B. Calculation of tooth size-jaw size discrepancies
C. Evaluation of cranio-facio-dental relationships
D. All of the above

Answers

1.A. Cephalometric evaluation helps in monitoring the growing developments during treatment and also helps in the assessment of post-treatment stability.

2.A. ANB angle indicates the horizontal relationship between maxilla and mandible. A positive value indicates a forward positioned maxilla, i.e. Class II pattern .

3.D. The cephalostat maintains a constant and reproducible spatial relationship with respect to the position of the patient's head, the film and X-ray source.

4.C. The film size of 25 × 20 cm(8 × 10 in) is used. The film is placed as close as possible to the patient's head.

5.B. Although A point may change with treatment ,it represents the most forward point of the maxilla.

6.B. Pogonion is the most anterior point on the mid-sagittal mandibular symphysis.

7.A. Basion is the most inferior posterior point on the occipital bone that corresponds to the anterior margin of the foramen magnum.

8.A. Frankfort horizontal plane represents the basic horizontal plane of the head.

9.D. Facial plane is a line constructed through the Nasion (N) perpendicular to the Frankfort horizontal plane.

10.C. Normal value of ANB angle is +2°.

11.C. Maxillary incisor angulations is the angle formed by the SN plane and the upper central incisor long axis.

12.D. Various workers such as Tweed, Down, Steiner , Holdaway, Bjork, Rakosi and Ricketts have given their cephalometric analysis based on different theories.

13.B. Facial angle determiner if the skeletal Class II or a Class III relationship is attributable to a retrognathic or a prognathic mandible.

14.D. The main goal of cephalometric analysis is to localize malocclusion within a geometric tracing of facial bone and soft tissue structure.

20

Preventive and Interceptive Orthodontics

1. Preventive dentistry is defined as:
  A. The correction of presently existing oral diseases to prevent their complications in the future
  B. The philosophy of dental practice dedicated to the prevention of all dental diseases
  C. The regular use of a selected series of procedures for the prevention of dental disease
  D. None of the above

2. Assessment of crowding in mixed dentition can be done by:
  A. Observing the erupting permanent incisors
  B. Radiographic examination
  C. Mixed dentition analysis
  D. All of the above

3. In compensating extraction:
  A. The tooth is extracted but not necessarily contralateral tooth of the same arch
  B. The tooth extracted is of the same side but of the opposing arch to equalize drift in the two arches
  C. Tooth is extracted before the completion of root formation
  D. None of the above

4. For the prevention of distal drift of permanent incisors:
  A. Space maintainers are used
  B. Balancing extraction is preferred
  C. Both of the above
  D. None of the above

5. What is the cause of Midline diastema?
  A. Supernumerary tooth **B.** High frenum attachment
  C. Mesiodens **D.** All of the above

6. Closure of midline diastema by moving two central incisors towards each other is an example of:

A. Reciprocal anchorage
B. Muscular anchorage
C. Intermaxillary anchorage
D. No anchorage

7. Effect of premature loss of a tooth in a child is:

A. Change in occlusion
B. Development of abnormal oral habits
C. Disturbed phonetics
D. All of the above

8. Premature exfoliation of a primary mandibular canine is most often the sequela of which of the following?

A. Caries
B. Trauma
C. Serial tooth extraction
D. Arch length inadequacy

Answers

1.B. Preventive orthodontics includes space control, space maintenance, space regaining, functional analysis and oral habit check up, muscle exercises, prevention of Milwaukee brace damage, etc.

2.D. Mixed dentition analysis is a part of preventive dentistry. It is done to foresee the problem of crowding in permanent dentition.

3.B. In balancing extraction, the tooth extracted is generally, but not necessarily, contralateral tooth of the same arch.

4.B. Space maintainer is used to prevent the mesial drift of the permanent first molar. Space maintainers are not used to prevent the distal drift of permanent incisors because this only occurs if the incisors are crowded.

5.D. Midline diastema associated with heavy labial frenum can be treated by frenectomy.

6.A. Reciprocal anchorage is the form in which the resistance is offered by two malposed units, when the dissipation of equal and opposite forces tends to move each malposed unit towards each other to achieve normal occlusion.

7.D. Effect of premature loss of a tooth in a child is change in occlusion, development of abnormal oral habits and disturbed phonetics.

8.D. Premature exfoliation of the deciduous canine on the crowded side, due to a midline displacement of the permanent mandibular incisors is most often the sequela of true hereditary tooth size and jaw size discrepancy.

21

Serial Extraction

1. **Serial extraction is indicated primarily in:**
   A. Lower anterior crowding only
   B. Class II malocclusion
   C. Class III malocclusion
   D. Class I malocclusion

2. **Extraction of deciduous incisors:**
   A. Needs a space maintainer
   B. Enhances the possibility of protrusion
   C. Does not have any effect on the developing permanent dentition
   D. None of the above

3. **The treatment objective of serial extraction is:**
   A. To direct eruption of permanent teeth in a favorable position and direction
   B. Reduce appliance treatment time
   C. Reduce the discomfort to the patient
   D. All of the above

4. **Planned and sequential removal of deciduous and permanent teeth is known as:**
   A. Balanced extraction
   B. Compensating extraction
   C. Serial extraction
   D. None of the above

5. **Serial extraction is indicated:**
   A. When tooth size, arch length discrepancy is less or equal to 5 mm
   B. When tooth size, arch length discrepancy is equal or less than 7 mm
   C. When tooth size, arch length discrepancy is equal or more than 7 mm
   D. None of the above

6. Better prognosis can be obtained by serial extraction in:
- **A.** Class I malocclusion
- **B.** Class II malocclusion
- **C.** Class III malocclusion
- **D.** None of the above

7. Ideal condition for serial extraction is:
- **A.** When age of patient is 7 to 8 years
- **B.** A true, relatively severe hereditary tooth-size jaw-size discrepancy is present
- **C.** Minimum overjet relationship of the incisor teeth
- **D.** All of the above

8. Which of the following is the sign of a true hereditary tooth-size jaw-size discrepancy:
- **A.** Maxillary and mandibular alveolo dental protrusion without inter proximal spacing
- **B.** Crowded mandibular incisor-teeth without interdental spacing
- **C.** Ectopic eruption of the permanent maxillary first molars, causing the premature exfoliation of the primary second molar
- **D.** All of the above

9. Which of the following is a contraindication of serial extraction?
- **A.** Class I malocclusion where the space deficiency is less than 7 mm and only slight crowding is present
- **B.** Congenital absence of any tooth except 3rd molar
- **C.** Deep overbite or excessive open bite
- **D.** All of the above

10. The preferred sequence of serial extraction can be:
- **A.** C-D-4
- **B.** D-4-C
- **C.** C-D-4 to D-4-C
- **D.** None of the above

11. Which of the following has poor prognosis for serial extraction?
- **A.** Class I malocclusion
- **B.** Class II malocclusion
- **C.** Dental Class III malocclusion
- **D.** Skeletal Class III malocclusion

12. In serial extraction procedures, concerns about the eruption sequence are usually related to the eruption pattern of which permanent teeth?

A. Maxillary canines and first premolars
B. Mandibular first and second premolars
C. Mandibular first molars and incisors
D. Mandibular canines and first premolars

Answers

1.D. Better prognosis can be obtained by serial extraction in Class I malocclusions because the dentition is basically in a favorable relationship and successful treatment is possible with a minimum of mechanotreatment.

2.C. Extractions of deciduous incisors do not have any effect on the developing permanent dentition. But extractions of deciduous canines and molars have definite effect on developing permanent incisors.

3.D. The treatment objective for serial extraction is to direct eruption of permanent teeth in a favorable position and direction, reduce malposition of teeth, reduce appliance treatment time, the cost of treatment and discomfort to the patient .

4.C. By this proper alignment of permanent teeth can be obtained whenever an arch length discrepancy is diagnosed at any early stage.

5.C. Serial extraction is indicated when it is ascertained "with certainty that there will not be sufficient space in the jaws to accommodate all the permanent teeth in their correct alignment".

6.A. Better prognosis can be obtained by serial extraction in Class I malocclusions because the dentition is basically in a favorable relationship and successful treatment is possible with a minimum of mechanotreatment .

7.D. Ideal conditions for serial extraction also include minimal overbite, a facial pattern that is orthognathic or with a slight alveolodental protrusion is present and crowding in deciduous dentition .

8.D. The true hereditary crowding is treated with the help of extraction, and if discovered early, with serial extraction, while crowding resulting form environmental factors may be treated without extractions.

9.D. Contraindications of serial extraction also include Class II division 2, Class III, skeletal malocclusion and excessive spacing .

10.C. Depending on the respective positions of the developing permanent teeth to the alveolar margin and on their inclination to prevent impaction of the first premolar, the sequence of serial extraction can be changed advantageously from C-D-4 to D-4-C .

11.D. Children with skeletal Class III malocclusion have poor prognosis for serial extraction .

12.D. Serial extraction procedure was first described by Robert Bunon in 1743.The term serial extraction was given by Kjellgran in 1929 .

22

Space Maintainers and Space Regainers

1. **Removable space maintainer has a disadvantage that it:**
   - **A.** May not be worn
   - **B.** Will not maintain horizontal dimension
   - **C.** Will not maintain vertical dimension
   - **D.** Cannot be made esthetic

2. **Requirement of space maintainer is:**
   - **A.** It should maintain the entire width of the space left by a missing tooth
   - **B.** It should prevent supraeruption of opposing tooth
   - **C.** It must restore function as far as possible
   - **D.** All of the above

3. **Indication of a removable space maintainer is:**
   - **A.** When esthetics is an important consideration
   - **B.** When more than two deciduous molars are missing
   - **C.** When more than one deciduous tooth is missing bilaterally
   - **D.** All of the above

4. **Which of the following is not a contraindication of a removable space maintainer:**
   - **A.** Uncooperative patients
   - **B.** Patients allergic to acrylic materials
   - **C.** Epileptic patients having uncontrolled seizures
   - **D.** None of the above

5. **Advantage of fixed space maintainer is:**
   - **A.** Minimum or no tooth preparation is required
   - **B.** It does not hamper the growth of jaws
   - **C.** The successive permanent teeth are free to erupt into the oral cavity
   - **D.** All of the above

6. Disadvantage of fixed space maintainer is:

I. Their construction needs elaborate instrumentation with expert skill

II. Decalcification of the tooth material may result under the bands

III. If pontics are not used, supraeruption of opposing teeth may take place

IV. They hamper the growth of jaw

A. I and II
B. I and III
C. I, II and III
D. All of the above

7. Most commonly used space maintainer is:

A. Band and loop space maintainer
B. Band and bar type
C. Distal shoe type
D. None of the above

8. Lingual arch space maintainer is used in:

A. Upper arch only
B. Lower arch only
C. Upper and lower arch
D. None of the above

9. Nance holding arch is used in:

A. Mandible
B. Maxilla
C. Both the mandible and maxilla
D. None of the above

10. Distal shoe space maintainer is used when:

A. The deciduous first molar is prematurely lost before the eruption of the permanent first molar
B. The deciduous second molar is lost before the eruption of permanent 1st molar
C. The anterior tooth is lost
D. All of the above

11. During the mixed dentition stage, which of the following appliances should be used as a space maintainer for missing primary molars in the mandibular arch?

A. Distal shoe
B. Nance holding arch
C. Passive lingual arch
D. Removal acrylic arch

12. **Most important factor in planning for a space maintainer is:**
    - **A.** Age of child
    - **B.** Amount of bone covering erupting permanent tooth
    - **C.** Stage of development of permanent tooth
    - **D.** Economical factors

13. **Distal shoe appliance is contraindicated in patients with:**
    - **A.** Congenital heart diseases
    - **B.** Hemophilia
    - **C.** Poor oral hygiene
    - **D.** All of the above

14. **All of the following are true of band and loop space maintainer except they:**
    - **A.** Are non-functional
    - **B.** Require less chair side time
    - **C.** Are removed and polished every year
    - **D.** Prevent over eruption of opposite teeth

Answers

1.A. Removable space maintainer has a disadvantage that uncooperative patients may not wear the appliance or they may be lost or broken by the patient.

2.D. Space maintainer is a device placed within the dental arch to prevent adjacent teeth from moving into the space left by a missing tooth .

3.D. Removable space maintainers can be removed and reinserted by the patient . They may be functional and non functional .

4.D. Functional space maintainers incorporate teeth to aid in mastication, speech and esthetics, whereas non functional space maintainers have only an acrylic extension over the edentulous area to maintain the space.

5.D. Minimum or no tooth preparation is required as bands and crowns are used .

6.C. Fixed space maintainers do not hamper the growth of jaw.

7.A. Band and loop space maintainer is a unilateral fixed appliance.

8.B. Lingual arch space maintainer is usually indicated in case of multiple loss of deciduous molars.

9.B. Nance holding arch is used in maxillary dental arch to prevent mesial migration of maxillary molars.

10.B. This appliance is used to guide the eruptive path of first permanent molar to the normal position.

11.C. Lingual arch space maintainer not only prevents mesial drifting of molars but also prevents lingual collapse of the anterior teeth.

12.B. Amount of bone covering the unerupted tooth aids in evaluating the probable time of eruption of the succedaneous tooth .

13.D. Medically compromised patients like patients with congenital heart diseases, kidney problems, juvenile diabetes, history of rheumatic fever and hemophilia, are contraindications of distal shoe appliance.

14.D. Band and loop space maintainer will not prevent the continued eruption of the opposing teeth . Decalcification under the bands is also a problem.

23

Oral Habits and their Management

1. **Harmful oral habits in children include:**
   A. Finger or thumb sucking
   B. Bruxism and mouth breathing
   C. Cheek, lip and nail biting
   D. All of the above

2. **Cribs can serve:**
   A. To make the habit nonpleasurable for the patient
   B. To remind the patient that he is indulging in the habit
   C. To break the suction and force on the anterior segment
   D. All of the above

3. **The oral screen:**
   A. Allows the passage of air through the mouth and nares
   B. Allows for the passage of air through the mouth
   C. Causes the child to breathe through the nose
   D. Prevents the passage of air through the nares

4. **Bruxism:**
   A. The etiology is epilepsy
   B. Is due to gastrointestinal disease
   C. The etiology is obscure
   D. The etiology is not obscure

5. **At some time thumb sucking is noted in:**
   A. All
   B. Over 50%
   C. 10 to 50%
   D. under 10%
   – of preschool children

6. **How long should a palatal crib be worn by a patient being treated for thumb sucking?**
   A. One month
   B. Three months
   C. Six months to one year
   D. Two to three years

7. Children suck their thumb or finger:
 A. When they are hungry
 B. When they are afraid
 C. After taking food
 D. All of the above

8. Thumb sucking habit is considered normal upto:
 A. 1–2 years of age
 B. 2–5 years of age
 C. 2½–3 years of age
 D. 5–6 years of age

9. Effect of thumb sucking on the maxilla is:
 A. Open bite with increased proclination of maxillary incisors
 B. Arch length of maxilla is increased
 C. Overjet is increased and the overbite is decreased
 D. All of the above

10. Effect of thumb sucking on the mandible is:
 A. Lingual inclination of mandibular incisors
 B. Labial inclination of mandibular incisors
 C. Arch length is increased
 D. Mandibular intermolar distance is decreased

11. Due to the habit of mouth breathing:
 A. Lower lip becomes hypoactive
 B. Lower lip becomes hyperactive
 C. Both lips become hypoactive
 D. Upper lip becomes hyperactive

12. Management of thumb sucking habit:
 A. Should be started at the age of 4 years
 B. Should be started at the age of 6 years
 C. Should be started at the age of 8 years
 D. Should be started at the age of 10 years

13. Management of thumb sucking habit is done by:
 A. Psychological approach
 B. Chemical approach
 C. Mechanical aids
 D. All of the above

14. Etiology of mouth breathing is:
A. Rhinitis and sinusitis
B. Over eruption of lower anterior teeth touching the palatal mucosa
C. Reduced size of airway due to deviated nasal septum
D. All of the above

15. Clinical feature of mouth breathing is:
A. Pigeon face appearance
B. 'V' shaped upper arch
C. Short and flaccid upper lip
D. All of the above

16. Effect of long-term tongue thrusting is:
A. Proclination of anterior teeth
B. Bimaxillary protrusion
C. Posterior cross bite
D. All of the above

17. Bruxism is seen in:
A. Chorea
B. Epilepsy
C. G.I.T. disturbances
D. All of the above

18. In cases of bruxism, the appliance usually given in childhood is:
A. Activator (Passive)
B. Hawley's appliance
C. Bite plate
D. Bionator

Answers

1.D. Harmful oral habits are frequent manipulation of lips, tongue or cheeks in a wrong manner with a variation from their normal use.

2.B. The most common professional method of treatment of thumb sucking has been the use of a palatal crib extending over the palatal arch preventing thumb sucking and setting in a negative behavior.

3.C. Mouth breathing can be checked by use of vestibular (oral) screen.

4.C. Bruxism is defined as non functional grinding or gnashing of the teeth.

5.C. Thumb sucking is observed slightly more in girls. It is seen at a younger age and is most common habit in infants.

6.C. The treatment can be successful only if the child is ready to help himself.

7.D. Children also suck their thumb or finger during stressful conditions .

8.C. Persistence of this habit beyond 3½ years of age can have a damaging influence on the dentoalveolar structures and should be intercepted.

9.D. Effect of thumb sucking on mandible are lingual inclination of mandibular incisors, increased mandibular intermolar distance and increased distal position of B point .

10.A. Thumb sucking also results in risk of speech defect deformation of digits and unilateral or bilateral class II malocclusion .

11.B. Mouth breathing also results in shortening and hypotonicity of upper lip.

12.A. The most common professional method of treatment by pedodontists and orthodontists has been the use of a palatal crib extending over the palatal arch preventing thumb sucking and setting in a negative behavior.

13.D. It is often seen that children lacking parental care, love, affection resort to this habit. Thus, the parents should be advised to provide the child with adequate love and affection

14.D. Mouth breathing may be obstructive or habitual in nature. Obstructive mouth breathing persists as a habit after the removal of the nasal obstruction .

15.D. Contraction of maxillary dental arch results in a V-shaped arch and high vault palate.

16.D. Tongue thrusting is an immature way of swallowing .

17.D. Chorea is ceaseless occurrence of rapid, jerky, dyskinetic, involuntary movements.

18.B. For the patients suffering from emotional or psychological disturbances, psychiatric help may be initiated.

24

Myofunctional Treatment

1. **Which of the following is not mainly a myofunctional appliance?**
   A. Inclined plane B. Activator
   C. Hawley's D. Oral screen

2. **The appliance which also acts as a lip bumper is:**
   A. Bionator B. Harvold's appliance
   C. Bimler's appliance D. The Kinetor

3. **Which of the following is not an indication for use of the activator?**
   A. Class I open and deep bite
   B. Class III malocclusion
   C. Post-treatment retention
   D. Excessive lower facial height

4. **Which of the following is not a contraindication for the use of activator?**
   A. Excessive lower facial height
   B. Non-growing individuals
   C. Class II division 1 malocclusion
   D. Severely procumbent lower incisors

5. **Myotactic reflex occurs by the use of which of the following appliance:**
   A. Activator appliance B. Bionator's appliance
   C. Bimler's appliance D. Frankel's appliance

6. **Activator was first developed by:**
   A. Andresen and Haupl B. Balters
   C. Frankel D. Harvold

7. **Bionator was first developed by:**
   A. Andresen and Haupl B. Balters
   C. Frankel D. Harvold

8. **The bionator appliance is used for:**
   A. Open bite cases
   B. Class II division 1 malocclusion
   C. Class 1 malocclusion with narrow dental arch
   D. All of the above

9. **The most commonly used appliance for the treatment of Class II division 1 and division 2 malocclusion is:**
   A. FR 1c B. FR 2
   C. FR 3 D. FR 4

10. **Bimaxillary protrusion is treated by:**
    A. FR 1 B. FR 2
    C. FR 3 D. FR 4

11. **Lip bumper which is used to distalize molars utilizes:**
    A. Intermaxillary anchorage
    B. Extraoral anchorage
    C. Muscular anchorage
    D. Intra-oral anchorage

Answers

1.C. Myofunctional or functional appliances are appliances which activate the patient's own muscles to function in such a manner which is conducive to orodental health.

2.C. The Bimler appliance also acts as lip bumper as it holds the lip away from lower incisors and facilitates their proclination .

3.D. Activator is most efficient in mouths where there is no shortage of space and the teeth are well-aligned.

4.C. Activator is most commonly used in class II division 1 malocclusion.

5.A. Muscular reflex is activated by use of activator appliance.

6.A. The activator is derived from the original appliance designed by Andresen in Norway after World War I. It is also known as Andresen appliance.

7.B. The bionatar was evolved by Dr Balters in West Germany.

8.D. As bionatar does not affect speech , it can be worn during the day.

9.B. Initials FR stand for 'Functional Regulator'.

10.D. FR4 is used primarily for the correction of open bite and bimaxillary protrusions to a lesser extent .

11.C. In certain cases, the perioral musculature is used as resistance unit to aid in the movement of teeth. An example of muscular anchorage is the use of a lip bumper to distalize molars.

25

Fixed and Removable Appliances

1. **Anterior crossbites may be treated by means of:**
   A. The steel crown with inclined band
   B. The tongue blade
   C. The bite inclined plane
   D. All of the above

2. **Protruding upper teeth with spacing may be treated by means of:**
   A. Maxillary Hawley-type acrylic appliance
   B. Steel crown
   C. Tongue blade
   D. Bite plane

3. **Adam's cribs can fracture in use if:**
   A. The tags are too high on the bite
   B. The wire is too soft
   C. The base plate is too thick
   D. The arrowheads are too small

4. **Which type of orthodontic tooth movement occurs mainly with the removable appliance?**
   A. Bodily
   B. Tipping
   C. Rotation
   D. Torquing

5. **Which of the following is not a part of the removable appliance?**
   A. Base
   B. Fixation, e.g. clasps
   C. Active component, e.g. cantilever spring and screw
   D. Passive component, e.g. ligature wire

6. **Hawley's removable appliance is an example of:**
   A. Intermittent force
   B. Continuous force
   C. Interrupted force
   D. Both A and C

7. **Which of the following appliances does not use intra-oral anchorage?**
   A. Transpalatal bar
   B. Goshgarion's appliance
   C. Mandibular holding arch
   D. None of the above

Answers

1.D. Anterior cross-bite may be prevented by timely removal of the cause, e.g. extraction of primary canines may allow crowded incisor to erupt in normal alignment.

2.A. Class I type 2 malocclusion has procumbent and spaced upper incisors. They can be treated by simple Hawley's appliance with labial bow. If initiating cause is any oral habit then it should be corrected.

3.A. Tags should be placed at the end of the retentive arms for retaining the clasp securely in the acrylic base.

4.B. In tipping type of tooth movement when force is applied to the crown, it results in movement of the crown in the direction of the force and root movement in the opposite direction.

5.D. The mechanical removable appliance consists of three parts: (i) the base, (ii) the fixation, (iii) the active component .

6.A. Intermittent force is applied for a short time and then released. Intermaxillary elastics, tooth positioners, headgears and the Hawley's removable appliance are typical examples of intermittent force.

7.D. In cases of intraoral anchorage, resistant units are all situated within the oral cavity.

26

Orthodontic Tooth Movement and Cross-bites

1. **Transposition is a condition:**
   A. Where two teeth of a same quadrant change position
   B. Where two teeth of the other quadrant change position
   C. Where two teeth of the other arches change position
   D. None of the above
2. **During orthodontic tooth movement at the site of pressure:**
   A. Bone resorption takes place
   B. Bone apposition takes place
   C. Cellular activity is increased
   D. Both A and C
3. **During orthodontic tooth movement at the site of tension:**
   A. Bone apposition takes place
   B. Cellular activity is increased
   C. There is formation of immature, poorly calcified bone trabeculae
   D. All of the above take place
4. **The orthodontic tooth movement in which the crown moves in the direction of the force and the root in opposite direction is called as:**
   A. Root torque
   B. Bodily movement
   C. Tipping
   D. Rotation
5. **Movement of root without movement of crown is known as:**
   A. Uprighting
   B. Root torque
   C. Bodily movement
   D. Tipping

6. The amount of force needed for interrupted force is:
- A. 200 to 300 gm 24 hours a day
- B. 200 to 300 gm 10 to 14 hours a day
- C. 110 to 200 gm 24 hours a day
- D. 300 to 500 gm 10 to 14 hours a day

7. Class II elastic traction between lower molars and upper anteriors is an example of:
- A. Mechanical anchorage
- B. Reciprocal anchorage
- C. Muscular anchorage
- D. Baker's anchorage

8. Posterior—cross-bite can be corrected by:
- A. Coffin spring
- B. Palatal Jack screw expansion appliance
- C. Quad helix spring
- D. All of the above

Answers

1.A. Transposition or transversion is a wrong sequential order. Here the teeth appear to have exchange places during the development of occlusion.

2.A. Bony tissue reacts to force for tooth movement by transforming into bone resorption and decreases the cellular activity at the site where pressure is applied .

3.D. Mild or light force can be applied at sporadic intervals to permit new osteoid tissue to develop in periods between appliance adjustments. It keeps the teeth firm and relatively pain free.

4.C. A typical example of tipping is to close anterior diastema and reduce the overjet in Class I malocclusion by removable Hawley's appliance.

5.B. Torquing can be considered as movement of the root in this type of tooth movement , the crown is held in position and the root is moved in a labial or lingual direction.

6.B. Interrupted force is an orthodontic or orthopedic force that is inactive for the interval of time between appointments.

7.D. The resistance units are situated in one jaw and are utilized to effect tooth movement in the opposing jaw are called intermaxillary anchorage. It is also called baker's anchorage.

8.D. Individual posterior cross bite is treated with removable appliance in which jack screw is inserted in the palatal acrylic, buccal movement of the maxillary posterior teeth will occur. Care must be taken not to use excessive force, which may devitalize the tooth being moved.

27

Isolation of Teeth

1. Isolation of teeth is done for:
   (i) Dry and clean field
   (ii) Better access and visibility
   (iii) Prevention of interference from other structures such as lips, cheek and tongue
   (iv) Getting improved properties of dental materials and better results
   (v) Protection of patient and operator
   A. (i), (ii) and (v) only
   B. (i), (ii) and (iii) only
   C. (i), (ii), (iii) and (v) only
   D. All of the above

2. Ideally isolation of teeth is brought about by:
   A. Rubber dam
   B. Cotton rolls
   C. Absorbent wafers
   D. Suction devices

3. Rubber dam cannot be used for following conditions:
   (i) Partially erupted teeth
   (ii) Extremely malposed and tilted teeth
   (iii) Attrited teeth
   (iv) Allergy to rubber dam material
   A. (i) and (ii) only
   B. (i), (ii) and (iii) only
   C. (i), (ii) and (iv) only
   D. All of the above

4. Thickness of rubber dam ranges from:
   A. 0.006 to 0.030 inch
   B. 0.006 to 0.014 inch
   C. 0.006 to 0.2 inch
   D. 0.012 to 0.2 inch

Answers

1.D. Purpose of the isolation of teeth is for preventing the infection and injury to other structures of oral cavity of the patient during the operation.

2.A. Ideally isolation is brought about by the use of rubber dam. Secondly, we can use cotton rolls, absorbent wafers and suction devices and drugs.

3.C. Rubber dam also can't be used in asthmatic patient's and mouth breathers.

4.B. Thick sheet causes more gingival retraction but tears less.

28

Pit and Fissure Sealants

1. **For partially erupted permanent molars the appropriate sealant is:**
   A. Glass ionomer cement
   B. Dimethacrylate
   C. Polyurethane
   D. Cyanoacrylate

2. **For fully erupted teeth the appropriate sealant is:**
   A. Glass ionomer cement
   B. Dimethacrylate
   C. Polyurethane
   D. Cyano-acrylate

3. **The visible light curing sealants are sensitive in the wavelength region of:**
   A. 580 nm
   B. 470 nm
   C. 310 nm
   D. 750 nm

4. **Retention of fissure sealants is chiefly the result of which of the following?**
   A. Mechanical microretention
   B. Adhesion of the sealant
   C. Chemical bonding of the sealant with the enamel
   D. Physical penetration of the sealant into the pits and fissures

Answers

1.A. An application of fissure sealant without acid etching on the enamel surface of a partially erupted tooth is a clinically acceptable and effective procedure in caries prevention .

2.B. In 1965 Bowen and associates had developed bisGMA resin, which is the chemical reaction product of bisphenol A and glycidyl methacrylate.

3.B. The visible light curing sealants have diketones and aromatic ketones, which are sensitive to visible light in the wavelength region of 470 nm (blue region).

4.A. 25 to 50 mm of enamel surface is rendered porous by the acid solution. It is into this porous region that the resin is able to penetrate and so bond with the enamel.

29

Fluoride and Dental Health

1. After topical fluoride treatment:

A. The child must not eat, drink or rinse his mouth for at least half an hour

B. The child must not rinse his mouth with water

C. The child can eat and drink, but should not rinse his mouth for at least half an hour

D. Once the fluoride has been applied, it doesn't make any difference what touches the tooth surface

2. Recommended dose of fluoride in drinking water is:

A. 0–0.5 ppm B. 0.5–1.0 ppm

C. 1.0–1.5 ppm D. 1.5–2.0 ppm

3. Average lethal dose of fluoride for adults is:

A. 2–4 gm B. 5–6 gm

C. 8–10 gm D. 1–2 gm

4. Average lethal dose of fluoride for infants is:

A. 0.1–0.2 gm B. 0.2–0.3 gm

C. 0.3–0.4 gm D. 0.4–0.5 gm

5. Drinking water which has more than following concentration must be defluoridated:

A. 5 ppm fluoride B. 2 ppm fluoride

C. 3 ppm fluoride D. 4 ppm fluoride

6. Using topical fluoride, caries can be inhibited up to:

A. 50% B. 70%

C. 90% D. 100%

7. How much concentration of sodium fluoride is used in prevention of caries by topical application?

A. 1% B. 2%

C. 8% D. 10%

8. How much concentration of SnF_2 is used in prevention of caries?

A. 2% B. 4%
C. 6% D. 8%

9. Systemic administration of fluoride is done by:

A. Fluoride gels, solutions and varnishes
B. Mouth rinses
C. Water fluoridation
D. All of the above

10. Which of the following is not a systemic effect of fluoride?

A. Renders the enamel more resistant to acid dissolution
B. Inhibition of bacterial enzymes
C. Modification of the size and shape of teeth
D. Reduced tendency of plaque formation

11. Artificial water fluoridation was first started in:

A. New York
B. Grand Rapids town in Michigan
C. Paris
D. Blue cross town in UK

12. Compounds used for milk fluoridation are:

A. Calcium fluoride
B. Disodium monofluorophosphate
C. Disodium silicofluoride
D. All of the above

13. Which of the following statements is inappropriate?

A. Fluoride absorption from milk is the same as that from water
B. Sodium fluoride is the most extensively used agent for large scale fluoridation
C. Amount of fluoride added in milk depends upon the age of the child and fluoride concentration in water
D. None of the above

14. Topical application of sodium fluoride (Knutson's technique) is done at the ages of:

A. 4, 8, 10 and 13 years
B. 3, 7, 10 and 13 years
C. 3, 7, 11 and 13 years
D. 3, 7, 11 and 15 years

15. The pH and fluoride concentration of APF gel and solution is:

A. 3 and 1.23%
B. 3 and 2.23%
C. 4 and 2.23%
D. 4 and 1.23%

16. Role of calcium carbonate, calcium phosphate, silicon oxide, aluminium oxide and granular polyvinyl chloride in a dentifrice is to:

A. Reduce calculus deposition
B. Clean the tooth mechanically
C. Help in the removal of loose debris
D. All of the above

17. Fluoride level in excess of following leads to staining of teeth:

A. 2 ppm
B. 3 ppm
C. 4 ppm
D. 5 ppm

18. Dental fluorosis occurs in the permanent dentition only. It can be prevented by restricting children's intake of fluoride during the enamel calcification period:

A. Both statements are TRUE
B. Both statements are FALSE
C. The first statements is TRUE, the second is FALSE
D. The first statement is FALSE, the second is TRUE

19. The children in an elementary school exhibit a high interproximal caries rate. Which of the following school-based programs will be MOST effective?

A. Sealant
B. Fluoride mouthrinse
C. Brushing and flossing
D. None of the above

20. If a child is born and has lived for first eight years in area which contains water supply with 2.5 ppm of fluoride, mottling develops:

A. In all primary teeth
B. In all permanent teeth
C. In all permanent teeth except third molars
D. Only permanent incisors are affected

Answers

1.A. This prolongs the availability of fluoride ion to react with the tooth surfaces.

2.B. 0.5 to 1ppm fluoride is most cost effective with a minimum of undesirable effects (fluorosis).

3.D. Lethal dose of fluoride depending on the body weight for adults is 3 to10 gm (average 5 to 6 gm).

4.D. Lethal dose of fluoride depending on the body weight for infants is 0.25 to 0.8 gm (average 0.4 to 0.5 gm).

5.A. Defluoridation of water means the downward adjustment of the level of fluoride content of drinking water supply to an optimal level just enough to prevent caries and not to cause fluorosis of bone and teeth .

6.B. Topical fluoride therapy means the local or topical application of relatively high concentration of fluoride to all erupted surfaces of teeth to prevent dental caries.

7.B. Bibby 1941 and Knutson 1942, 1947 and 1948 have used various concentration and frequencies of application in various studies. They concluded that 2 percent solution should be applied and allowed to dry on the surfaces of teeth for a few minutes.

8.D. Stannous fluoride solution should be freshly prepared from stannous fluoride packed in a prefilled "O" No. gelatin capsule (an airtight container) in order to prevent oxidation of salt.

9.C. Systemic administration also include salt fluoridation, flour fluoridation , milk fluoridation, fluoride supplements in the form of tablets, drops and lozenges.

10.D. Systemic effects of fluoride also includes reduction of enamel tendency to absorb protein.

11.B. In 1945, artificial water fluoridation was carried out in a town Grand Rapids in Michigan. This was the first city in the world to have artificial water fluoridation.

12.D. Sodium fluoride has been the most extensively used agent for large scale milk fluoridation.

13.D. Milk fluoridation involves the addition of a fluoride compound to milk in the appropriate quantity such that the resultant product contains the fluoride concentration in the required amount.

14.C. 2 percent sodium fluoride solution should be applied and allowed to dry on the surfaces of teeth for a few minutes. This is performed once a week for four consecutive weeks at the ages of 3,7,11 and 13 years.

15.A. APF gel can be self applied by children under supervision, by using self reusable or disposable trays in various sizes, together with sponge-like tray liners.

16.B. Detergents like sodium lauryl sulfate and sodium-N-lauryl sarcosinate in 1 to 5 percent help in the removal of loose debris.

17.C. The optimum fluoride level of 1ppm in drinking water is absolutely safe and useful for caries prevention.

18.D. During maturation period of enamel maximum fluoride is taken up by the enamel. Therefore, the maximum advantage of fluoride application will take place during this maturation period of enamel.

19.B. 0.05 percent sodium fluoride solution used daily as a mouthwash is more effective in preventing caries, than fluoride dentifrices.

20.C. Drinking water having more than 5 ppm fluoride must be defluoridated.

30

Anesthesia During Management

1. **What type of drug is usually used to eliminate pain?**
   A. Anesthetic B. Sedative
   C. Narcotic D. Analgesic

2. **For dental treatment, general anesthesia is indicated in:**
   A. In an uncooperative child where all conventional management procedures have failed
   B. In severely handicapped children
   C. In child with severe congenital heart disease
   D. All of the above

3. **Extraction in general anesthesia is performed when:**
   A. The patient is uncooperative
   B. There is allergy to local anesthetic solution
   C. Both of the above
   D. Teeth should not be extracted under general anesthesia

4. **During injection technique of local anesthesia to minimize pain:**
   A. The anesthetic solution should be warmed up to body temperature
   B. A topical local anesthesia should be applied at the site of the injection
   C. Anesthetic solution should be injected slowly
   D. All of the above

5. **In children when giving inferior alveolar nerve block, the level of needle should be lower as compared to adults (S). It is because the height of ramus in children is less than adults (R):**
   A. Both 'S' and 'R' are removed
   B. 'S' is true while 'R' is false
   C. 'S' is false while 'R' is true
   D. Both 'S' and 'R' are false

6. **Which of the following is not a complication that may arise after administration of local anesthesia?**
   A. Vomiting
   B. Ulcer on lip
   C. Herpetiform lesion
   D. None

7. **What determines the maximum dose of local anesthesia for a child?**
   A. Age
   B. Weight
   C. The procedure to be accomplished
   D. The desired degree of pulpal anesthesia

Answers

1.D. The control of pain while performing dental procedures for the child is one of the most fundamental and important components which supports the sound principles of behavior management.

2.D. The drug for general anesthesia can be administered by any of the parenteral route. But before giving anesthesia, patient's medical history must be taken and family physician should be contacted.

3.C. General anesthesia is a drug which induced loss of consciousness during which patients are not arousable, even by painful stimulation accompanied by complete loss of protective reflexes.

4.D. The disadvantage with topical anesthetics is that they have disagreeable taste, but nowadays few flavored topical anesthetics are also available.

5.A. The inferior alveolar nerve is to be blocked when operative or surgical procedures are to be done for mandibular primary or permanent teeth.

6.D. Maximum dose of lidocaine without vasoconstrictor is equal to weight of the patient × 4 mg/kg, and with vasoconstrictor is equal to weight of the patient × 6 mg/kg.

7.B. The potential for anesthetic toxicity is increased when local anesthetics are used in young patients, who are sedated with medications before the treatment.

31

Heredity in Pedodontics

1. **Hereditary hypohydrotic ectodermal dysplasia is manifested by:**
   A. Hypohidrosis B. Hypotrichosis
   C. Hypodontia D. All of the above

2. **In majority of the cases the ectodermal dysplasia is:**
   A. Sex linked recessive
   B. Sex linked dominant
   C. Autosomal dominant
   D. Autosomal recessive

3. **"Thistle tube" appearance is seen in:**
   A. Radicular dentin dysplasia
   B. Coronal dentin dysplasia
   C. Dentinogenesis imperfecta
   D. Ectodermal dysplasia

4. **Which of the following statements is not true about dentinogenesis imperfecta?**
   A. It is also termed as opalescent dentin
   B. Type I always occurs in families with osteogenesis imperfecta
   C. Both dentitions are equally affected in Type I whereas deciduous teeth are more severely affected in Type II
   D. Type III has same clinical appearance of teeth as Type I and Type II but also has multiple pulp exposure

5. **Amelogenesis imperfecta mainly is:**
   A. Autosomal dominant
   B. Autosomal recessive
   C. Sex linked recessive
   D. Sex linked dominant

6. **In hereditary vitamin D resistant rickets:**
   A. There is high blood alkaline phosphatase level and hypophosphatemia
   B. The pulp chamber and root canal appear large radiographically
   C. The dentin is poorly calcified
   D. All of the above

7. **Ectodermal dysplasia is characterized by:**
   A. Hypodontia
   B. Hypotrichosis
   C. Hypohidrosis
   D. All of the above

8. **Severe form of erythema multiforme is known as:**
   A. Stevens - Johnson syndrome
   B. Peutz-Jeghers syndrome
   C. Down's syndrome
   D. Albright's syndrome

Answers

1.D. In this syndrome there are abnormalities of skin, hair, nails, eyes, teeth, facies and sensorineural apparatus in various combination and varying severity.

2.A. But sometimes it may be as straight dominant character. The skin of the patient is soft and smooth, thin, dry with partial or complete loss of sweat glands.

3.B. The permanent tooth exhibits an abnormally large pulp chamber in coronal portion of tooth roentgenographically and this is called "Thistle-tube" appearance.

4.C. In general the deciduous teeth are more severely affected in type I and in Type II, both dentitions are affected equally.

5.A. The amelogenesis imperfecta is a group of hereditary defects of enamel unassociated with any other generalized defects.

6.D. Hereditary vitamin D resistant rickets condition is transmitted as a sex-linked dominant characteristic.

7.D. Hereditary hypohydrotic ectodermal dysplasia is a specific syndrome characterized by congenital dysplasia of one or more ectodermal structures and their accessory appendages, manifested by hypohydrosis, hypotrichosis and hypodontia

8.A. Stevens-Johnson syndrome is a severe form of erythema multiforme involving fever and lesions of the oral, conjuctival and vaginal mucous membrane and marked by a cutaneous rash that is often widespread and severe.

32

Restoration of Deciduous Teeth

1. The following factors must be considered before restoring a deciduous tooth:

A. Degree of carious involvement
B. Time of normal exfoliation and space consideration in the arch
C. Age of the child
D. All of the above

2. Acid etching of deciduous teeth is done for:

A. 30 to 60 seconds
B. 60 to 90 seconds
C. 90 to 120 seconds
D. 120 to 150 seconds

Answers

1.D. In primary teeth, the cavity preparation is smaller due to smaller crown size, shallower due to thin enamel and narrower due to narrow occlusal table.

2.C. Etching of deciduous teeth does not produce a good retentive surface due to the larger amount of exogenous organic material found in deciduous enamel, i.e. prism less layer resulting from its lower mineral content.

33

Amalgam and Composite Restorations

1. **Before amalgam is inserted into any cavity:**
   A. The area should remain dry during the entire insertion and carving procedure
   B. Pulpal wall should not be flat or smooth
   C. The area should not be clean
   D. Occlusal enamel wall should not be parallel to axis tooth

2. **Poorly condensed and contaminated amalgam has the following features:**
   A. Faltering margins
   B. Blistering
   C. Marked expansion
   D. All of the above

3. **Big amalgam filling after few years often tends to discolor the tooth. This can be prevented by using:**
   A. Rubber dam
   B. Zinc-free alloy
   C. Cavity varnish on all cut surfaces of cavity before filling
   D. Calcium hydroxide on the pulpal floor

4. **Should low copper amalgam be burnished after carving?**
   A. No, it brings mercury to the surface of the margin
   B. Yes, it makes the surface look shiny
   C. Yes, it continues condensation at the margins
   D. No, it might destroy the crystal structure

5. **Ideal isthmus width for Class II cavity preparation for silver amalgam should be:**
   A. ½ of the dimension between the buccal and lingual cusps
   B. ¼ of the dimension between the buccal and the lingual cusps
   C. ⅓ of the dimension between the buccal and lingual cusps
   D. ⅓ to ¼ of the dimension between the buccal and the lingual cusps

6. **Matrix band adaptation is:**
   - **A.** Difficult in permanent as compared to the deciduous teeth
   - **B.** Difficult in deciduous as compared to the permanent teeth
   - **C.** Same in both the cases
   - **D.** Cannot say

7. **Amalgam restoration with high mercury content shows:**
   - **A.** Greater frequency of surface roughness
   - **B.** Less frequency of surface roughness
   - **C.** Less frequency of marginal breakdown
   - **D.** None of the above

8. **Tensile strength of the amalgam can be improved by:**
   - **A.** Increasing the tin content
   - **B.** Decreasing the tin content
   - **C.** By increasing the Hg content
   - **D.** Decreasing the Hg content

9. **The range of dimensional change upon setting in the case of silver amalgam is:**
   - **A.** –10 to +10 mm/cm **B.** 0 to +10 mm/cm
   - **C.** 0 to +20 mm/cm **D.** –20 to +20 mm/cm

10. **For the acid etching of the tooth surface:**
    - **A.** 30 to 50% phosphoric acid is applied for 40 seconds
    - **B.** 40 to 60% phosphoric acid is applied for 40 seconds
    - **C.** 30 to 50% phosphoric acid is applied for 60 seconds
    - **D.** 40 to 60% phosphoric acid is applied for 40 seconds

11. **If the viscosity of the resin is increased:**
    - **A.** It will reduce penetration of resin into acid etched enamel
    - **B.** It will increase penetration of resin into acid etched enamel
    - **C.** It will have no effect on penetration of resin
    - **D.** Cannot be predicted

12. **Coupling agents are used:**
    - **A.** Before the acid etching
    - **B.** After the acid etching
    - **C.** After the application of bonding agents
    - **D.** None of the above

13. **Which material is used as a base in composite resin?**
    - **A.** Zinc phosphate **B.** Polycarboxylate
    - **C.** Glass ionomer cement **D.** None of the above

14. Which of the following statements is correct for composite resin?

A. $Ca(OH)_2$ can be used as a base material
B. ZnOE interferes with the curing process of composite resin
C. Cavity varnishes alter the hardness of the composite resin
D. All of the above

15. Which of the following statements is correct?

A. Deciduous teeth should be etched for more time than permanent teeth to produce equal etching.
B. Surface of deciduous teeth contains more exogenous organic material than does the surface of permanent teeth
C. Acid softened enamel can reharden in presence of saliva
D. All of the above

Answers

1.A. The effect of moisture contamination during condensation process reduces the compressive strength of amalgam, restoration, causing a delayed expansion of the amalgam.

2.D. Proper condensation is important for marginal adaptation, corrosion resistance, smooth polished surface and maximum strength.

3.C. The application of two or three thin layers of quick drying varnish to freshly cut dentin will also reduce sensitivity after the placement of the filling.

4.C. Carving should be done using sharp instruments and with strokes either proceeding from tooth surface to amalgam surface or laterally along tooth amalgam interface. However high capper amalgam does not show improvement with burnishing.

5.D. Isthmus is the narrowest part of the occlusal outline near the proximal box.

6.B. The matrix should be rigid enough to allow adequate packing pressure without deformation, ensuring a well condensed filling which, is free from an excess of residual mercury.

7.A. The mercury concentration is characteristically higher in the marginal areas than the body or bulk of the restoration.

8.B. The strength of amalgam depends upon the mercury content present in amalgam (from about 42 to 64 percent) and the tensile strength of the amalgam may be improved by decreasing the tin content.

9.D. During setting, contraction or expansion is characteristic of dental amalgam.

10.C. The acid etched enamel surface should have a matte appearance. If the viscosity of the resin increases then it reduces penetration of the resin into acid etched enamel.

11.A. Etching increases surface area by forming pores into which resin can flow resulting in mechanical retention.

12.B. Coupling agents have been used with composite resins to further enhance the composite adhesion to tooth structure.

13.D. Cavity varnishes have also been reported to react at the interface of restoration and alter the hardness of the composite resin.

14.D. The composite resins irritate the pulpal tissue due to the presence of methacrylate monomers as diluents in the composite. Due to this reason, when dentin is exposed and a composite restoration is placed, pulp protection should be done.

15.D. The etched enamel surface has a high surface energy and allows the resin to readily wet the surface and penetrate into the microporosities.

34

Atraumatic Restorative Treatment

1. **Full form of ART is:**
   A. Automatic restorative therapy
   B. Automatic restorative treatment
   C. Atraumatic restorative treatment
   D. Atraumatic restorative therapy

2. **Which of the following instruments is not required in the ART?**
   A. Excavator
   B. Dental hatchet
   C. Carver
   D. Burs

3. **Which of the following is done in atraumatic restorative procedure?**
   A. Glass ionomer cement restoration
   B. Self-cure resin composite restoration
   C. Indirect pulp capping procedure
   D. All of the above

Answers

1.C. Atraumatic restorative treatment (ART) is a new procedure which consists of manually cleaning dental cavities with hand instruments and filling them with an adhesive and fluoride releasing material.

2.D. Easily available inexpensive hand instruments are used rather than the expensive electrically driven dental equipment.

3.D. Indirect pulp capping procedure involves removal of gross carious lesion and sealing of cavity with a dentinogenesis promoting bactericidal agent for four to six weeks.

35

Tooth Colored Restorative Materials and Cements used in Pedodontics

1. **Silicate cements are contraindicated for children:**
   A. Who brush their teeth three times daily
   B. Who are mouth breathers or have protruding incisors
   C. Who drink fluoridated water
   D. None of the above

2. **The most commonly used castable ceramic is:**
   A. Cerestore B. Dicor
   C. Bonded alumina D. All are equally used

3. **Adaptation of resin can be improved by the use of:**
   A. Cavity liners
   B. Acid etching technique
   C. A and B both
   D. None. The resins are directly applied

4. **The commonly used coupling agents in filled or conventional composite resin is:**
   A. Titanates and Zirconates
   B. Quartz
   C. Barium and strontium
   D. Triethylene glycol

5. **In light activated resins, which chemical is added as inhibitor in order to prevent or minimize spontaneous polymerization of monomer:**
   A. Triethylene glycol
   B. Titanates and Zirconate
   C. Colloidal silica
   D. Butylated hydroxy toluene

6. **The particle size of macrofilled composite resin is:**
   A. More than 200 microns
   B. 10 to 100 microns
   C. 1 to 10 microns
   D. 0.1 to 1 micron

7. **The particle size of minifilled composite resin is:**
   A. 1 to 10 microns
   B. 0.1 to 1 micron
   C. 0.01 to 0.1 micron
   D. 0.001 to 0.01 micron

8. **The degree of polymerization within the bulk of the photo initiated resin depends upon:**
   A. The thickness of filling
   B. The intensity of light beam
   C. The number, size and distribution of the filler particles
   D. All of the above

9. **Medium fusing dental porcelain has fusion temperature between:**
   A. 1300 to 500°C B. 1101 to 1300°C
   C. 850 to 1100°C D. 700 to 850°C

10. **Which of the following is an advantage of acid-etch technique prior to cementation?**
   A. Increases surface area
   B. Creates the micromechanical bonding of the composite cement to ceramic restoration
   C. Better retention
   D. All of the above

11. **Light cured lining glass ionomer cements are classified as:**
   A. Type I B. Type II
   C. Type III D. Type IV

12. **Restorative glass ionomer cement is classified as:**
   A. Type I B. Type II
   C. Type III D. Type IV

13. **Fusion of the glass powder with sintered silver particles by high temperature fusion is:**
   A. Cermet B. Dicor
   C. Inceram D. Optec-Hsp

14. Resin modified glass ionomer cement is called as:
A. Cermet
B. Inceram
C. Dicor
D. Compomer

15. The weakest cement is:
A. Zinc phosphate
B. Zinc oxide eugenol
C. Calcium hydroxide
D. Silicate cement

16. Calcium hydroxide cement is used in:
A. Pulpotomy
B. Apexification
C. As an intracanal medicament
D. All of the above

17. Light cured resins use:
A. Magnetochromic light
B. UV light
C. Visible light
D. Both B and C

18. Function of coupling agent in restorative resin is to allow:
A. Bonding between filler and resin
B. Bonding between tooth and resin
C. Bonding between filler crystals
D. All of the above

19. Which of the following contains anticariogenic property:
A. Glass ionomer cement
B. Silicate cement
C. Both A and B
D. None

Answers

1.B. Silicate cement use has been almost discontinued as it gives rise to adverse pulpal reactions because of low pH.Other disadvantages include erosion , sensitivity and dimensional instability due to shrinkage solubility in oral fluids.

2.C. DICOR is a castable glass that is formed into an inlay facial veneer or full crown restorations by the lost wax casting process.

3.C. Etching of deciduous teeth does not produce a good retentive surface due to the large amount of exogenous organic material found in deciduous enamel, i.e. prism less layer resulting from its lower mineral content.

4.A. Coupling agents bond the filler particles to the resin matrix. These agents improve the physical and mechanical properties and provide hydrolytic stability by preventing water penetration along filler resin interface .

5.D. Inhibitor like 0.01 wt percent of butylated hydroxytoluene is added to resin in order to prevent or minimize spontaneous polymerization of monomer.

6.B. Macrofilled composite resin is no longer used because of poor properties and are called conventional or traditional. The most commonly used filler is ground quartz.

7.B. The particle size of microfilled composite resin is 0.01 to 0.1 micron.

8.D. The degree of polymerization within the bulk of the photo initiated resin also depends upon the translucency of the resin.

9.B. Medium fusing dental porcelain are used for fabrication of artificial denture teeth

10.D. Acid etching strengthens previously weakened tooth structure by bonding ceramic restoration to the acid etched enamel surface.

11.C. The already shrunken precured glass ionomer particle are blended into composites so as to increase strength and to reduce overall total shrinkage.

12.B. Restorative glass ionomer cements are of two type, i.e. Class 1 esthetic restorative cements and Class 2 reinforced restorative cements or metal modified glass ionomers.

13.A. Mixing of spherical silver amalgam alloy powder with glass ionomer powder. This mixture is referred to as silver alloy admix or miracle mix.

14.D. The word compomer derives its name from the hybridization of composites and glass ionomers, i.e. Composite + Glass Ionomer =Compomer.

15.B. Zinc oxide eugenol cement has bacteriostatic property.

16.D. Commercially available calcium hydroxide products are dycal, life, pulpdent, etc.

17.C. Light cured composites are available as a single paste in syringe . The initiating system consists of the photo-initiator molecule and an amine activator.

18.A. Coupling agents improve the physical and mechanical properties and provide hydrolytic stability by preventing water penetration along filler-resin interface.

19.C. In glass ionomer and silicate cements, anticariogenic environment is established due to constant leaching of fluoride from the materials.

36

Pediatric Endodontics

1. **After a partial pulpectomy has been completed, the permanent restoration ideally should be placed:**
   - **A.** At the same appointment
   - **B.** After six weeks when a radiograph indicates no bone destruction between the roots
   - **C.** After approximately two weeks after making certain the tooth is comfortable
   - **D.** After six months when a radiograph shows bonds of calcification across the root canals
2. **During initial stage of pulpal pathology localization of pain is:**
   - **A.** Relatively simple to determine
   - **B.** Extremely difficult
   - **C.** Cannot be explained by psychophysiology
   - **D.** Depends upon the intensity of the stimulus
3. **In indirect pulp capping the medicament of choice is:**
   - **A.** Zinc oxide and eugenol
   - **B.** Zinc oxide and thymol
   - **C.** Zinc oxide and eucalyptol
   - **D.** Calcium hydroxide
4. **The simplest form of pulp therapy is:**
   - **A.** Apicoectomy
   - **B.** Pulp capping
   - **C.** Pulpotomy
   - **D.** Pulpectomy
5. **Partial pulpotomy is:**
   - **A.** Removal of entire coronal pulp
   - **B.** Pulp capping
   - **C.** Enlargement of carious exposure and placement of medication
   - **D.** None of the above

6. **Anterior deciduous teeth:**
   A. Are the best candidates for endodontic treatment
   B. Are poor risks for endodontic treatment
   C. Contain ribbon-like root canals
   D. Contain tortuous and multifurcated root canals

7. **Direct pulp capping is indicated:**
   A. When there is small traumatic exposure (1 mm or less) of a vital pulp
   B. In carious exposures with completed root formation
   C. For any case of pulp exposure since it is 100 percent successful
   D. None of the above

8. **The following represent/s possible treatment plans for the tooth with an exposed pulp:**
   A. Extraction of the tooth
   B. Pulp capping
   C. Pulpectomy (total removal of pulp)
   D. All of the above

9. **A nonvital deciduous maxillary lateral incisor with pulpal abscess in a 5-year old patient should be treated by:**
   A. Pulpectomy
   B. Wait and watch the child at regular intervals
   C. Extraction
   D. Formocresol pulpotomy

10. **The treatment of choice for a deciduous tooth having recent mechanically exposed pulp is:**
    A. Calcium hydroxide pulpotomy
    B. 5-minute formocresol pulpotomy
    C. 7-day formocresol pulpotomy
    D. Pulpectomy

11. **Calcium hydroxide applied in indirect pulp capping procedures should remain for at least:**
    A. 5 minutes
    B. 6 to 8 weeks
    C. 4 to 6 months
    D. 1 to 2 weeks

12. During the root canal treatment procedure of the deciduous tooth, injury to the permanent tooth bud can cause:

A. Hypocalcification of permanent tooth
B. Hypodysplasia of permanent tooth
C. Dilaceration of the permanent tooth
D. All of the above

13. Contraindication of direct pulp capping is:

A. Pulp exposure of more than 2 mm in diameter
B. Carious exposure surrounded by infected dentin
C. Pulpal pathology
D. All of the above

14. Pulpotomy is a process in which:

A. Only radicular pulp is removed
B. Only coronal pulp is removed
C. Whole pulp is removed
D. None of the above

15. Contraindication to pulpotomy is:

A. Pulp calcifications
B. Profuse hemorrhage from the exposure site
C. Tenderness to percussion
D. All of the above

16. Which of the material is used in pulpotomy in deciduous teeth?

A. Calcium hydroxide
B. Formocresol
C. Glutaraldehyde
D. All of the above

17. Which of the following materials is used for obturation of deciduous teeth?

A. Gutta percha B. $Ca(OH)_2$
C. Silver nitrate D. Iodoform paste

18. Contraindication for deciduous root canal filling is:

A. Teeth with mechanical/carious perforations of the floor of the pulp chamber
B. Excessive pathologic root resorption
C. The presence of dentigerous/follicular cyst
D. All of the above

19. Which of the following instruments should be used to prepare the canals of deciduous teeth?
A. Reamers and files
B. Gates Glidden drill
C. Sonic and ultrasonic cleaning devices
D. Any of the above

20. Which of the following materials is used for obturation of deciduous teeth?
A. Walkoff's paste
B. PD Iodoform paste
C. Cresopaste
D. All of the above

21. Which one of the following is a disadvantage of gutta-percha when used as a root canal filing material ?
A. Lack of rigidity in thinner size
B. Biocompatibility
C. Solubility in organic solvent
D. All of the above

22. By which route pulpal inflammation reaches the periodontal area?
A. Accessory canals B. Through apical foramina
C. Furcation D. All of the above

23. Which of the following tooth shows maximum number of endodontic treatment failures?
A. Maxillary lateral incisor
B. Maxillary second premolar
C. Mandibular first premolar
D. None of the above

24. A cooperative 5-year-old child has a carious lesion in her primary mandibular second molar. There is no tooth mobility, but the practitioner notes a small, draining sinus tract adjacent to the tooth. Which of the following is the treatment-of choice?
A. Extraction
B. Pulpectomy
C. Indirect pulp therapy
D. Formocresol pulpotomy

25. Which of the following best describes the radiolucency seen at the furcation of the mandibular right second primary molar?

A. It is of pulpal origin
B. It is of periodontal origin
C. It is of combined pulpal and periodontal origin
D. It is a normal feature of the mixed dentition

26. Cotton pellet applied to the pulpal stumps after formocresol pulpotomy should be:

A. Dampened with formocresol
B. Saturated with formocresol
C. Left in place for 5 minutes
D. Left in place until second visit

27. Chronic pulpal infection in primary molars is first noticed radiographically:

A. As internal resorption
B. As rarefaction of periapical tissues
C. As rarefaction at bony furcation
D. As widening of periodontal space

Answers

1.C. Partial pulpectomy is performed in primary teeth when both the coronal and only cervical one-third of the radicular pulp tissues show clinical evidence of infection.

2.B. Deciduous teeth with a history of spontaneous unprovoked toothache should be considered for pulp capping , pulpotomy or pulpectomy.

3.D. Calcium hydroxide in a methyl cellulose and metacresyl acetate base is shown to produce bridging of regular reparative dentin.

4.B. Often young vital teeth have not fully completed their root formation .Therefore, the prime requisite is to maintain the integrity of radicular pulp. To achieve this goal, as far as possible, techniques of vital pulp treatment should be employed.

5.D. The only difference between pulpotomy and pulp capping is that in pulpotmy, all coronal pulp tissue is removed from the exposed pulp and in pulp capping no pulp tissue is removed.

6.A. In very small and uncooperative children , the nonvital pulpotomy technique is often used even for a tooth with a necrotic pulp, though pulpectomy may be attempted if the condition are favorable. These difficulties do not exist with deciduous anterior teeth and, therefore, pulpectomy of these teeth presents no technical problem.

7.A. Direct pulp capping involves the application of a medicament or dressing to the recently exposed pulp with very small pin point sized exposure in an attempt to preserve its vitality.

8.D. Extraction is preferable to pulp treatment if the opposite molar is missing and cannot be replaced.

9.A. Deciduous teeth are the best natural space maintainer.

10.B. Formocresol solution releases formaldehyde, which diffuses through the pulp and combines with cellular protein and fixes the tissue. The fixed tissue may later become replaced by vital granulation tissue.

11.B. Dentin is laid down fastest during the first month following indirect pulp capping .The rate than diminishes steadily with time.

12.D. Fear of damage to developing permanent tooth buds and a belief that the tortuous root canals of deciduous teeth cannot be adequately negotiated , cleaned , shaped and filled have led to the needless sacrifice of many pulpally involved deciduous molars.

13.D. Other contraindications include teeth with history of spontaneous pain and excessive bleeding indicating hyperemia or pulpal inflammation.

14.B. Pulpotomy can be defined as surgical amputation of the coronal pulp followed by placement of a suitable medicament over the radicular tissue, in order to promote healing .

15.D. Any signs and symptoms which suggest that inflammation has extended beyond the coronal pulp into root canals is a contraindication to pulpotomy.

16.D. Because of mutagenic and carcinogenic potential of formocresol many workers support the use of glutaraldehyde instead of formocresol for pulpotomy.

17.D. The filling material for deciduous root canals must be resorbable, so that it is resorbed along with the roots and dose not interfere with the eruption of the permanent teeth .

18.D. Other contraindications include a nonrestorable tooth, radiographically visible internal resorption in the roots, excessive pathologic loss of bone support with loss of the normal periodontal attachmant.

19.A. Only very thin files and reamers of short length should be used. These short length endodontic instruments are specially designed for child patients.

20.D. The iodoform paste is bactericidal to microorganisms in the root canals and loses only 20 percent of its potency over a period of 10 years .

21.A. Gutta percha is difficult to introduce into a narrow root canal, and it does not seal a canal apically or laterally unless it is combined with root canal cement or sealer. Gutta percha has a limited shelf life, it becomes brittle with age .

22.D. The presence of patent lateral or accessory canals is an important factor in the development of pulpoperiodontal disease of the individual tooth .

23.C. Various reasons of failure are inaccessible lateral (accessory) canal, broken instrument or other cause of blockage of canal, perforation, inadequate instrumentation, inadequate sterilization, inadequate obturation, severe periodontal involvement communicating with a root canal.

24.B. Pulpectomy is performed in primary teeth when both the coronal and radicular pulp tissue show clinical evidence of infection.

25.A. Evidence that the floor of the pulp chamber is perforated due to caries, internal resorption or mechanical instrumentation is radiographic contraindication for endodontic therapy.

26.A. In young permanent teeth with incompletely developed root apices, evidence of continued root development following formocresol pulpotomy procedure has been observed .

27.C. Recent radiographs (periapical and bitewing) are essential for examining the extent of caries and changes in periapical tissues.

37

Management of Immature Permanent Tooth

1. **Root canal treatment cannot be done in immature permanent tooth because:**
   A. Radicular pulp is not well developed
   B. Root is not completely formed
   C. Root apex is wide
   D. Working length cannot be measured

2. **Blunderbuss apex is:**
   A. Apex covered by pathology
   B. Wide open apex
   C. Apex restricted by pulp stone
   D. Fractured apex

3. **Apexification is the process done in:**
   A. Vital pulp in young immature tooth
   B. Non vital pulp in young immature tooth
   C. Both of the above
   D. None of the above

4. **Mostly used material for the apexification is:**
   A. $Ca(OH)_2$
   B. Camphorated paramono chlorophenol
   C. Cresanol
   D. Metacresyl acetate

5. **Time required to achieve apexification is:**
   A. 2 to 6 months
   B. 6 to 12 months
   C. 6 to 24 months
   D. 12 to 24 months

6. **Which of the following is a disadvantage of apexification:**
   A. Successful rate of apexification is very low
   B. Such tooth is prone to fracture
   C. Both of the above
   D. None of the above

7. Loss of pulp vitality before the root length completion causes:

A. Poor crown to root ratio
B. Tooth being more prone to fracture
C. Problem in endodontic treatment
D. All of the above

Answers

1.C. In immature permanent teeth root- apex is so wide that root canal treatment cannot be done because of inability to condense gutta percha point or any other root canal obturating material. These wide open apices are called "blunderbuss apices .

2.B. Management of these teeth is a challenging task which requires patience, time, clinical skill and judgement.

3.B. Apexification process is also called as root end induction.

4.A. Calcium hydroxide alone or in combination with antibacterial drugs has become the most widely accepted material to promote apexification.

5.C. Patient is recalled at 3 months interval for monitoring the tooth.

6.C. The most important factors in achieving apexification seem to be proper debridement of the root canal and sealing of the tooth to prevent the ingress of bacteria and substrate.

7.D. Loss of pulp vitality before the root length completion causes poor crown to root ratio, tooth being more prone to fracture and problem in endodontic treatment.

38

Traumatic Injuries to the Teeth and Supporting Structures in Children

1. **The tooth most frequently involved in a traumatic episode is the:**
   A. Mandibular lateral incisor
   B. Mandibular central incisor
   C. Maxillary central incisor
   D. Maxillary lateral incisor

2. **The incidence of trauma to the anterior teeth of children is:**
   A. Increasing
   B. Decreasing
   C. Remaining essentially constant
   D. None of the above

3. **There is a real relationship between the incidence of fractured anterior teeth and the:**
   A. Protrusion of those teeth
   B. Hardness of the dentin
   C. Hardness of the enamel
   D. Caries in those teeth

4. **The most common cause of trauma to the anterior teeth of children is:**
   A. Accidents in the school yard
   B. Games
   C. Thrown stones
   D. Drinking at the fountain or from soda bottles

5. **Among fractures of anterior teeth, the incidence of fractures to teeth in the maxilla is:**
   A. 75 percent **B.** 25 percent
   C. 90 percent **D.** 50 percent

6. **The commonest fracture of Class I to the anterior teeth of children is:**
   A. Labial surface only
   B. The distoincisal angle
   C. Gingival third of tooth
   D. The mesioincisal angle

7. **Immediate treatment for Class I fracture of permanent teeth of children includes:**
   A. Placing mix of zinc oxide and eugenol on rough edges of enamel
   B. Elimination of the rough edges of enamel which abrade the tongue and protect exposed dentin with varnish
   C. Varnish rough edges of enamel
   D. Cement orthodontic band on tooth

8. **In most of the cases following tooth displacement, the periodontal fibers:**
   A. Are only stretched
   B. Are never lacerated
   C. Are unaltered
   D. Show stretching with laceration of fibers, apical vessels and nerves

9. **Immediate treatment for the intruded type of displacement is:**
   A. Place orthodontic appliance on tooth
   B. Extract tooth
   C. Warm saline washes and watchful waiting
   D. Withdraw the tooth into normal position

10. **What is the most frequent cause of failure of cases of replantation?**
    A. Ankylosis
    B. Internal resorption
    C. External resorption
    D. Pulp necrosis

11. **Peak incidence period for dental injuries is:**
    A. 1 to 2 years of age
    B. 2 to 3 years of age
    C. Young school age
    D. Mixed dentition age

12. The most susceptible age for the injury to the anterior permanent dentition is:
A. 8 to 10 years
B. 10 to 12 years
C. 12 to 14 years
D. 14 to 16 years

13. Maxillary central incisors are affected in about:
A. 50% of the total tooth injuries
B. 75% of the total tooth injuries
C. 80% of the total tooth injuries
D. 90% of the total tooth injuries

14. Ellis and Davey have classified injures to tooth and soft tissues into:
A. Six classes
B. Seven classes
C. Eight classes
D. Nine classes

15. Ellis classified injuries of tooth and soft tissues into:
A. Six classes
B. Seven classes
C. Eight classes
D. Nine classes

16. According to Ellis and Davey, in Class 5 fracture:
A. Traumatized tooth becomes non vital with or without loss of crown structure
B. Teeth lost as a result of trauma
C. Fracture of root
D. Displacement of a tooth without fracture of crown or root

17. WHO classification for injuries is for:
A. Deciduous teeth only
B. Permanent teeth only
C. Both deciduous and permanent teeth
D. None of the above

18. "Pink spot" is a sign of:
A. Internal bleeding
B. Necrotic pulp tissue
C. Internal resorption
D. External resorption

19. Which of the following statements is correct about external resorption?
A. It is usually seen where damage to the periodontal structure with some degree of tooth displacement occurs
B. Pulp is not involved and tooth is asymptomatic
C. In some cases, external resorption is arrested after some time
D. All of the above are correct

20. **Deep crazing and fracture lines on the enamel can be detected by:**
    A. Transillumination test
    B. Staining the teeth with a disclosing solution
    C. Radiographs
    D. All of the above

21. **Crazing of the enamel of the anterior teeth occurs due to:**
    A. Blow from a hard object
    B. Sudden change in temperature of tooth from very hot to very cold
    C. Excessive masticatory force
    D. All of the above

22. **According to the classification of root fracture, the Class 4 fracture is:**
    A. Fracture line below the gingival level but above alveolar crest level
    B. Fracture line with coronal third of root but below the level of alveolar crest
    C. Fracture line within middle third of root but below the level of the alveolar crest
    D. Fracture line in apical third of root

23. **According to the classification of the root fracture, the Class 3 fracture is:**
    A. Fracture line above gingival level
    B. Fracture line below the gingival level but above alveolar crest level
    C. Fracture line with middle third of root
    D. None of the above

24. **Management of Class 1 or Class 2 root fracture is:**
    A. Placing a layer of calcium hydroxide in between the fractured parts
    B. Tooth segments can be stabilized by splinting
    C. Tooth segment is stabilized by splinting after placing $Ca(OH)_2$ between the fractured parts
    D. Splinting done after root canal treatment

25. **Avulsed tooth should be replanted into the socket:**
    A. within 10 minutes B. within 20 minutes
    C. As early as possible D. within 40 minutes

26. Which of the following is a common cause of failure of replantation:

A. Pulp necrosis
B. Fracture of tooth
C. Root resorption
D. All of the above

27. If a case of an avulsed tooth is reported, the patient should be instructed to:

A. Keep the avulsed tooth in the open socket
B. Hold the tooth under tongue in the mouth
C. Keep the tooth in milk
D. Any of the above

28. If the tooth is received within 30 minutes of avulsion:

A. It should be replanted into the socket and splinting should be done
B. It should be replanted after immediate RCT
C. Tooth should be cleaned by antiseptic solution and replanted after RCT
D. None of the above

29. An average rate of reparative dentin formation is:

A. 1 micron per day
B. 1.2 micron/day
C. 1.4 micron/day
D. 2.0 micron/day

30. Management of internal resorption can be:

A. Immediate RCT
B. Observe with periodic radiograph
C. Extraction of tooth
D. None of the above

31. A child comes with Class I fracture of maxillary central incisor, with sufficient loss of tooth structure. Treatment should be:

A. Emergency root canal treatment
B. $Ca(OH)_2$ application followed by crown
C. Acid etch composite restoration
D. None of the above

32. Which of the following most often causes dental trauma involving the primary dentition of children aged 1½ to 2 ½ years?

A. Physical child abuse
B. Lack of parental supervision
C. Under developed motor coordination
D. High frequency of accident-prone profiles

33. Which of the following is occasionally the cause of yellowish discoloration in a primary vital maxillary incisor without any history of trauma?

A. Blood pigments
B. Pulp chamber calcification
C. Internal resorption
D. Pulp necrosis

Answers

1.C. They are affected in about 90 percent of the total tooth injuries.

2.A. The prognosis for success depends upon the time period elapsed between the injury and the treatment.

3.A. Incidence of fracture of anterior teeth was more with Angle's Class II division 1 type of malocclusion .

4.B. Peak incidence period for dental injuries is the young school age. In this age group, about 35 percent of the total dental accidents take place.

5.C. In case of permanent teeth , males are more prone than females to sustain dental accidents, the ratio being approximately 2:1.

6.B. The frequency of enamel and dentin fracture is more than fracture exposing the pulp or root fracture .

7.B. If fracture takes place in erupting teeth, wait for continued eruption of the teeth and other changes in the occlusion.

8.D. Displacement range from simple looseness to acute positional changes, intrusion and partial or complete avulsion.

9.D. In most of the cases the intruded teeth will re-erupt in six to eight weeks even if little of the crown is shown.

10.C. Replantation is the technique in which a tooth is reinserted into the alveolus after its loss or displacement by accidental means.

11.C. In this age group, about 35 percent of the total dental accidents take place.

12.A. In primary dentition ,only slight sex difference is there with boys being more prone.

13.D. The teeth most commonly involved in a dental accident are the maxillary central incisors.

14.C. Ellis and Davey in 1960 classified injuries to tooth and soft tissues into eight classes. Later on Class IX to XI, three more Classes were added. Class IX is traumatic injuries to deciduous teeth. Class X is cyclic incomplete dislocation of the tooth. Class XI is when enamel crack is present but fractured fragment is not separated, as underlined dentin is not fractured.

15.A. The original Ellis classification consists of six basic groups: (1) Enamel fracture (2) Dentine fracture without pulp exposure (3) Crown fracture with pulp exposure (4) Root fracture (5) Tooth luxation and (6) Tooth intrusion.

16.B. In Class 5 fracture, replacement of missing tooth is needed; a removable or bonded resin prosthesis is given followed by a fixed prosthesis at a later date.

17.C. WHO classification also include other injuries (laceration of soft tissues of oral cavity), fracture or comminution of the alveolar process of mandible or maxilla, fracture of the body of mandible or maxilla.

18.C. When the crown is affected the vascular tissue of the pulp shines through the remaining thin shell of the tooth and the condition is referred to as "Pink spot".

19.D. Peripheral root resorption may take place in cases of severe trauma.

20.D. In transillumination, patient is seated in a darkroom and sharp pointed light is placed lingual to the tooth inside the mouth and labial surface is examined from all angles through a thin roll of black paper.

21.D. To prevent the fracture of the tooth, masticatory stresses of the tooth should be lessened. To repair cracks, minute shallow filling can be done.

22.C. Class 4 root fracture is when the fracture line extends below the level of the alveolar crest, but within the middle third of the root. If the fragments are grossly displaced prognosis is poor.

23.C. Class 3 fracture is fracture line with coronal third of root but below the level of alveolar crest. Prognosis is favorable and fragments are not displaced.

24.C. In most of the cases it is difficult to stabilize the crown segment and prognosis for fracture repain is poor because bacteria and saliva infect the fractured area from the gingival crevice. After stabilization RCT is done. Intraradicular splinting is done or after removing. Coronal protein dowel (post and core) crown can be fabricated.

25.C. The success of treatment defends on the length of time for which, before transplantation, the tooth was out of the mouth, and the condition of the periodontal ligaments which are remaining on the surface of the root.

26.C If signs of root resorption or periapical inflammation are seen, root canal treatment should be done.

27.D. If the tooth is received within 30 minutes of avulsion, it should be replanted into the socket and splinting should be done. The prognosis will be better.

28.A. If the avulsed tooth is dirty, the root surface should be cleaned before replanting by any solution which is used for storing the avulsed tooth.

29.C. The rate decreases markedly after 48 days. Dentin is laid down fastest during the first month following indirect pulp capping.

30.A. If internal resorption is detected early the tooth may be retained by endodontic procedures.

31.C. If fracture is of long standing and the tooth is asymptomatic, good cosmetic results can be obtained by placement of composite restorative material.

32.C. When the child starts to crawl, stand or walk the injuries usually increase and are usually related to the lack of motor coordination.

33.B. In vital discolored teeth, occasionally discoloration occurs due to idiopathic pulpal recession. Such teeth remain vital. But usually display a yellow discoloration like pulpless tooth.

39

Management of Temporomandibular Joint Disorders and Injuries in Children

1. **The nerve supply to TMJ is:**
   A. Auriculotemporal nerve only
   B. Greater auricular and masseteric nerves
   C. Superficial temporal only
   D. Auriculotemporal and masseteric
2. **The symptoms of Myofacial Pain Dysfunction Syndrome are:**
   A. Pain or tenderness in TMJ and masticatory musculature
   B. Limited or irregular movement of mandible
   C. Clicking or popping noise
   D. All of the above
3. **Craniomandibular disorder is also known as:**
   A. Pierre-Robin syndrome
   B. Gardener's syndrome
   C. Costen's syndrome
   D. Peutz-Jegher's syndrome
4. **In TMJ dysfunction syndrome, which of the following drug is given to relieve early morning syndrome:**
   A. Aspirin **B.** Diazepam
   C. Paracetamol **D.** Nimesulide
5. **Which of the following is/are sign/s of success in TMJ treatment?**
   A. At least 12 mm of lateral movement
   B. Condyle is centered in fossa
   C. Condyle can translate past eminence with at least 2.5 mm distance between condyle and articular eminence
   D. All of the above

6. **The treatment of complete anterior dislocation of the meniscus, the procedure performed usually is:**
   A. Condylotomy and meniscal repair
   B. High condylectomy and meniscal repair
   C. Remedial exercises and heat treatment
   D. Any of the above

7. **Which of the following statements is false?**
   A. Rheumatoid arthritis affects women twice as much as men
   B. In most of the children having juvenile rheumatoid arthritis, TMJ is also involved
   C. In rheumatoid arthritis condyles and joint structures may be destroyed
   D. None

8. **To treat the dislocation of the joint, the pressure is applied:**
   A. Posteriorly and inferiorly
   B. Inferiorly and posteriorly
   C. Upwards and posterior
   D. Posteriorly only

Answers

1.D. The temporomandibular joint is a synovial joint of condylar variety.

2.D. The functional disturbances of TMJ are known by different names like "Costen's Syndrome", "TMJ dysfunction syndrome", "Myofacial pain dysfunction syndrome"., "Mandibular dysfunction" and "Craniomandibular disorders (CMD)",

3.C. The prevalence of TMJ dysfunction in childhood is high , only a few children with recurrent headache and frequent stomatognathic symptoms like reduced opening capacity of the mouth need treatment.

4.B. A night dose of diazepam 2 to 5 mg for two weeks relieves pain and early morning stiffness.

5.D. Other signs of success include no lateral deviation on opening or closing, at least 50 mm of mouth opening and no signs or symptoms on opening and closing.

6.B. A condylotomy is a procedure in which the condyle is removed or the neck of the condyle is surgically treated, usually allowing some forward and medial displacement of the condylar fragment.

7.D. There is no specific treatment for rheumatoid arthritis , although remarkable improvement may result from the administration of ACTH or cortisone . On total limitation of movement and deformity, condylectomy may be done to regain movement.

8.A. When the mouth is wide open , it is a sudden locking and immobilization of the jaws, accompanied by prolonged spasmodic contraction of the masticatory muscles.

40

Discolored Vital Tooth Bleaching and Laminated Veneers

1. **All discolored teeth are always:**
   A. A focus of infection
   B. Should be extracted
   C. Nonvital
   D. None of the above

2. **Pyrozone is very effective for bleaching discolored nonvital teeth. It consists of:**
   A. 25% hydrogen peroxide
   B. 25% ether
   C. One part chloroform and three parts ethyl alcohol
   D. 25% hydrogen peroxide in ether

3. **Bleaching in vital teeth cannot be done in:**
   A. Extremely large pulp horns
   B. Sensitive teeth
   C. Very dark teeth
   D. All of the above

4. **Walking bleach technique:**
   A. Is a heat treatment procedure
   B. Uses the mixture of sodium perborate and 35 % hydrogen peroxide
   C. Both of the above
   D. None of the above

5. **Which one of the following has maximum cleaning and bactericidal property in RCT?**
   A. Normal saline
   B. Formocresol
   C. Sodium hypochlorite
   D. Hydrogen peroxide

6. A permanent maxillary central incisor of a 12-year-old boy has become brown, yet the other teeth appear normal. This can be due to:
A. Tetracycline use
B. Exogenous staining
C. Traumatic injury to tooth
D. All of the above

7. Which of the following is not an external cause of tooth discoloration?
A. Tobacco chewing
B. Chromogenic bacteria
C. Cigarette smoking
D. Tetracycline

8. The cause of tooth discoloration in children is:
A. Tetracycline
B. Dentinogenesis imperfecta
C. Sickle cell anemia
D. All of the above

9. The material used for veneering is:
A. Composite
B. Porcelain
C. Cast cement materials
D. All of the above

10. In tetracycline discoloration, staining is usually present on:
A. Occlusal third of crown
B. Middle third of crown
C. Gingival third of crown
D. Whole surface of crown

11. The bleaching solution of vital teeth contains:
A. Anesthetic ether, hydrochloric acid and hydrogen peroxide
B. Anesthetic ether, superoxol and H_2O_2
C. Superoxol and anesthetic ether
D. 30% H_2O_2 and hydrochloric acid

12. For bleaching the vital teeth the hydrochloric acid is present in the concentration of:
A. 30% B. 36%
C. 40% D. 45%

13. For bleaching of vital teeth the hydrogen peroxide is present in the concentration of:

A. 20% B. 25%
C. 30% D. 35%

14. The bleaching solution for vital teeth contains anesthetic ether, hydrochloric acid and hydrogen peroxide in the ratio of:

A. 1: 1: 1 B. 1: 2: 4
C. 1: 5: 3 D. 1: 5: 5

15. The commonly used solution for night guard vital bleaching contains:

A. 30% H_2O_2
B. 10% H_2O_2
C. 10% carbamide peroxide
D. 30% carbamide peroxide

16. The common side effects of night guard vital bleaching are:

A. Tissue irritation on the gingival papilla
B. Gingival crest like a small burn or ulcer
C. Hypersensitivity to temperature changes
D. All of the above

17. A 6-year-old patient has a dark brown discoloration of his maxillary central incisor. The discoloration started following trauma accompanied with a labial sinus tract. What is the treatment of choice?

A. Extraction
B. Pulpectomy
C. Pulpotomy
D. Direct pulp treatment

18. A 5-year-old child received tetracycline therapy. Which of the following teeth may be affected:

A. Canines, premolars and second molars
B. First, second and third molars
C. Incisors and canines
D. All of the above

Answers

1.D. Discolored teeth can be divided into two types–(1) Discolored teeth with non-vital pulp or pulpless teeth and (2) Discolored teeth with vital pulp.

2.D. The goal of bleaching procedures is the restoration of normal color to a tooth by decolorizing the stain with a powerful oxidizing or reducing agent .

3.D. In vital discolored teeth, pulp is vital but discoloration occurs due to external causes.

4.B. Superoxol can be used alone or mixed with sodium perborate into a paste for use in the walking bleach. When sealed into the pulp chamber, it oxidizes and discolors the stain slowly, continuing its activity over a longer period of time. This procedure is called the "walking bleach".

5.C. Sodium hypochlorite vapors are bactericidal, whereas those of formocresol, aqueous para-chlorophenol are bacteriostatic.

6.C. Fresh supply of blood is cut off due to trauma leading to discoloration.

7.D. Other external causes of tooth discoloration include tobacco, medication , food and beverages.

8.D. All these are internal causes of tooth discoloration .

9.D. Veneers can be described as a layer of tooth colored material which is applied on the tooth surface for esthetic purpose.

10.C. Tetracycline discoloration is due to its use during pregnancy upto the age of 8 years.

11.A. 1 part of anesthetic ether, 5 parts of hydrochloric acid and 5 parts of hydrogen peroxide.

12.B. Hydrochloric acid etches the enamel .

13.B. Hydrogen peroxide bleaches the enamel.

14.D. Anesthetic ether removes surface debris and facilitates deeper penetration.

15.C. The night guard vital bleaching or matrix bleaching or "dentist-prescribed, home–applied" technique is easy and requires less "in office" time than other vital bleaching techniques.

16.D. If teeth become hypersensitive, the night guard is removed and bleaching is suspended or the exposure time is reduced, which alleviates the problem.

17.B. Pulpectomy is the removal of both coronal and radicular pulp.

18.A. The degree of staining and tooth stained depends on the stage of tooth development at the time when medication is taken. The greater the amount of crown developed, the less severe the stain, and vice versa .

41

Crowns in Pedodontics

1. **The following type/s of restoration can be placed where more then 80% crown of anterior tooth has been lost:**
   A. Fabricated acrylic jacket crown with post and core
   B. Preformed acrylic crown
   C. Stainless steel crown without labial window
   D. All of the above

2. **The factor/s which influence the design of crown is/are:**
   A. Extent of decay of tooth
   B. Periodontal health
   C. Occlusal forces
   D. All of the above

3. **Which of the following is not an indication for full coronal coverage of crown?**
   A. Teeth with poor interproximal contacts
   B. Discolored anterior teeth
   C. Teeth that have received pulp therapy
   D. None

4. **Porcelain jacket crown is given in:**
   A. Vital discolored teeth
   B. Teeth with poor interproximal contact
   C. Endodonticallly treated teeth
   D. Anterior teeth with multiple hypoplastic defect

5. **Which of the following is a contraindication for the polycarboxylate crowns?**
   A. Teeth affected with nursing bottle syndrome
   B. Discolored teeth
   C. Grossly broken teeth
   D. Root canal treated teeth

6. **Which of the following cements is not used for cementation of polycarboxylate crowns?**
   A. Zinc oxide eugenol cement
   B. A crown and bridge cement
   C. An acrylic cement only
   D. An acrylic intermediary followed by a crown and bridge cement

7. **The gingival margin for the stainless steel crown should be:**
   A. Knife-edge type
   B. Feather edge type
   C. Bevel type
   D. None

8. **The cements used for cementation of stainless steel crown to preparation are:**
   A. Zinc oxide eugenol
   B. Polycarboxylate
   C. Zinc silicophosphate
   D. All of the above

9. **The best cement for cementation of stainless steel crown is:**
   A. Zinc oxide eugenol
   B. Polycarboxylate
   C. Zinc silicophosphate
   D. Glass ionomer

Answers

1.A. Acrylic crown is cemented on the tooth with zinc phosphate cement.

2.D. The amount of occlusal forces brought to bear on a crown also modifies the crown design, increased occlusal forces are due to increased muscular activity and habit of bruxism.

3.D. Other indications for full coronal coverage of crown are teeth that have been fractured and have lost an appreciable amount of tooth structure, anterior teeth with multiple hypoplastic defect or developmental disturbance.

4.C. Porcelain jacket crown requires adequate tooth reduction for the strength of restoration.

5.C. Adequate retention cannot be obtained if tooth crown is badly destroyed.

6.A. Zinc oxide eugenol should not be used because the eugenol will soften and discolor the polycarbonate crown.

7.B. The gingival margin of the preparation, which is present on the proximal surface, should be smooth, feather edge with no ledge or shoulder present.

8.D. It is important to realize that when adapting stainless steel crowns, we prepare the tooth as per the crown, where as in a cast crown , we fabricate the crown according to the, tooth preparation.

9.D. Glass ionomer cements are the best cement for cementation of stainless steel crown because these cements release fluoride and chemically bond to the tooth structure.

42

Oral and Maxillofacial Surgery in Children

1. **Etiology of alveolar abscess is:**
   - **A.** Bacterial invasion by dead pulp tissue
   - **B.** Trauma
   - **C.** Mechanical or chemical irritation
   - **D.** All of the above
2. **Most common cyst of the jaws in children and adolescents is:**
   - **A.** Dentigerous cyst
   - **B.** Eruption cyst
   - **C.** Premordial cyst
   - **D.** Thyroglossal cyst
3. **Dentigerous cyst develops from:**
   - **A.** Rest cell of Malassez
   - **B.** Accumulation of fluid between the reduced enamel epithelium and enamel.
   - **C.** Degeneration of the enamel organ
   - **D.** None
4. **Premordial cyst develops from:**
   - **A.** Rest cell of Malassez
   - **B.** Accumulation of fluid between the reduced enamel epithelium and enamel.
   - **C.** Degeneration of the enamel organ
   - **D.** None
5. **The most common fissural cyst is:**
   - **A.** Nasopalatine duct cyst
   - **B.** Globulomaxillary cyst
   - **C.** Epidermoid cyst
   - **D.** Thyroglossal cyst

6. **In the radiological examination odontoma appears as:**
   A. Multilocular lesion
   B. Soap bubble appearance
   C. Irregular radio-opaque mass or small tooth structure
   D. None

7. **Which of the following is not a choice of treatment of ameloblastoma?**
   A. Cauterization
   B. Surgical excision
   C. Radiotherapy
   D. Chemotherapy

8. **Osteosarcoma is:**
   A. Two times more common in mandible
   B. Two times more common in maxilla
   C. Same in both
   D. Cannot predict

9. **Which of the following tumor is radio resistant?**
   A. Osteosarcoma
   B. Ameloblastoma
   C. Both of the above
   D. None of the above

10. **A purulent lesion in the facial vestibule of an 8-year-old child is mostly due to:**
    A. Pyogenic granuloma
    B. Odontogenic fistula
    C. Odontogenic tumor
    D. All of the above

11. **If during extraction of deciduous tooth, the permanent tooth bud comes out, then:**
    A. It should be placed back in the socket in bucco-lingual position and socket is sutured
    B. It should be thrown out
    C. Wash it properly, do pulpotomy and then place back
    D. None of the above

12. **The most commonly occurring impacted tooth in children is:**
    A. Mandibular canine
    B. Maxillary canine
    C. Mandibular IInd premolar
    D. Maxillary IInd premolar

13. **Ludwig's angina involves:**
   A. Submandibular and submental space only
   B. Submandibular and sublingual space only
   C. Submental and sublingual space only
   D. Submandibular, submental and sublingual space

14. **Commonest cause leading to Ludwig's angina is:**
   A. Carious exposed tooth
   B. Trauma in floor of oral cavity
   C. Jaw fracture
   D. Osteomyelitis

15. **The most common organism responsible for Ludwig's angina is:**
   A. *Streptococcus viridans*
   B. *Staphylococcus aureus*
   C. *Streptococcus hemolyticus*
   D. *Pseudomonas*

16. **Diagnosis of Ludwig's angina is made by:**
   A. Swelling in floor of oral cavity
   B. Tender bilateral swelling in submandibular, submental and sublingual regions
   C. Elevated tongue
   D. All of the above

17. **Commonest facial bone to fracture is:**
   A. Mandibular bone **B.** Nasal bone
   C. Zygomatic bone **D.** Maxilla

18. **The facial bones of children do not fracture easily because:**
   A. Maxillary sinus is poorly developed and ethmoidal and sphenoidal sinuses are not developed
   B. Bone is softer due to more organic content
   C. Condyle is not properly developed
   D. All of the above

19. **What would be the immediate concern of a dentist after removing the primary mandibular left second molar of a 3-year-old child?**
   A. Preventing lip biting
   B. Preventing a dry socket formation
   C. Controlling postoperative pain
   D. Preventing postoperative swelling

20. A healthy 3-year-old child has just had a routine extraction of a primary mandibular molar. Which of the following postoperative problems is the most likely to occur?

A. Prolonged bleeding
B. Pain
C. A dry socket
D. Lip bite

21. Best method to extract lower primary second molar to prevent injury to permanent tooth bud is to:

A. Luxate the tooth buccally
B. Luxate the tooth lingually
C. Luxate the tooth around long axis
D. Split the tooth and remove in two pieces

Answers

1.D. An acute alveolar abscess is a collection of pus in the alveolar bone at the root apex of a tooth following death of the pulp, with extension of the infection through the apical foramen into the periradicular tissue.

2.A. Dentigerous cyst is present adjacent to the crown of an unerupted tooth and attached at the C.E.J.

3.B. As it enlarges , epithelial lining gradually becomes stratified and may be carried away from the crown.

4.C. In primordial cyst , a cyst is formed instead of a tooth. The most common site is the posterior part of the mandible where, in place of a third molar, a primordial cyst is formed.

5.A. Fissural cysts are non-odontogenic cysts derived from epithelial remnants entrapped along lines of fusion or from embryologic defects.

6.C. The recommended treatment for an odontoma is conservative surgical extrusion, taking care to remove the surrounding soft tissue.

7.C. Treatment for ameloblastoma is surgical removal according to location, clinical and radiographic extent of the lesion. Recurrence rate is 55 to 90 percent.

8.A. Ostcosarcoma is an uncommon highly malignant primary tumor of bone that occurs between 10 to 25 years of age.

9.B. Ameloblastoma is usually a benign odontogenic locally invasive neoplasm of enamel forming cells and is persistent and aggressive in nature.

10.B. A purulent lesion in the facial vestibule of an 8 year old child is mostly due to odontogenic fistula.

11.A. Section of deciduous tooth is advised before extraction when permanent tooth bud is within the curved roots of deciduous tooth.

12.B. At the time of its eruption, adjoining teeth i.e. lateral incisor and first premolar have already erupted. Many times it has been observed that these teeth tilt and cause lack of space for erupting canine.

13.D. Ludwig 's angina is a severe cellulitis of the submandibular submental and sublingual space because of infection.

14.A. The teeth commonly involved are mandibular second and third molar.

15.C. Some other organisms like streptococcus viridans, staphylococcus aureus, spirochete, fusiform and coliform bacilli, pseudomonas and candida albicans may also be present .

16.D. Difficulty in eating , drinking and swallowing may be present. In severe cases, difficulty in breathing may be present.

17.A. The most common bone in facial region which fracture is mandible bone. Next to mandible bone is nasal bone.

18.D. Condyle is not properly developed so there are more chances of their crushing in comparison to fracture.

19.A. Some complications that arise after administration of local anesthesia are vomiting, ulcer on the lip because of biting when it is anesthetized and herpetiform lesion by disturbance in the trophic innervation.

20.D. Ulcer on the lip may appear because of biting when it is anesthetized.

21.D. Sinus tract associated with the deciduous teeth should not be curetted as it may cause damage of the permanent tooth bud in the socket.

43

Therapeutic Agents in Pedodontics

1. **Which is a suitable alternative antibiotic, when a child is sensitive to penicillin?**
   A. Tetracycline **B.** Ampicillin
   C. Sulfanilamide **D.** Erythromycin

2. **Which of the following is a third generation cephalosporin?**
   A. Cefazoline **B.** Cefuroxime
   C. Cefotaxime **D.** All of the above

3. **Penicillinase resistant penicillin is:**
   A. Phenoxymethyl penicillin
   B. Dicloxacillin
   C. Amoxicillin
   D. Ampicillin

4. **Which of the following antihistamines has/have a sedative effect?**
   A. Hydroxyzone **B.** Promethazine
   C. Diphenhydramine **D.** All of the above

5. **"Gray baby syndrome" is caused by:**
   A. Acetomenophins
   B. Chloramphenicol
   C. Pentobarbitol
   D. Phenylbutazone

6. **Which penicillin can be given orally?**
   A. Penicillin G
   B. Penicillin V
   C. Ampicillin
   D. Both Penicillin V and Ampicillin

7. **Which of the following is a common side effect of ampicillin?**
   A. Nausea **B.** Diarrhea
   C. Vomiting **D.** None of the above

8. **Which one of the following cephalosporins is contraindicated during pregnancy?**
   A. Cefazoline
   B. Cefuroxime
   C. Cefotaxime
   D. All of the above

9. **The most effective antibiotic in oral infection is:**
   A. Erythromycin
   B. Penicillin
   C. Clindamycin
   D. Tetracycline

Answers

1.D. Erythromycin is bacteriostatic and has same efficacy as oral penicillin in eradicating group Aβ-hemolytic streptcocci. It is a gastric irritant so tablets are enteric coated.

2.C. Cefotaxime is mainly effective against gram negative rod shaped bacteria. It is contraindicated during pregnancy.

3.B. Other pencillinase resistant penicillins are cloxacillins and oxycillin.

4.D. Benzodiazepines like diazepam and lorazepam also have sedative effect.

5.B. Liver in the children cannot properly metabolize the drug, hence chloramphenicol can produce "Gray body syndrome".

6.D. Penicillin V is acid resistant penicillin, can be given orally. It is effective against same bacterial spectrum as penicillin G.

7.B. Ampicillin is broad spectrum , acid resistant and bactericidal. It is ineffective against penicillinase producing strains.

8.C. Cefotaxime is third generation cephalosporin, mainly effective against gram negative rod shaped bacteria.

9.B. Penicillin acts by interfering with the biosynthesis of bactericidal cell wall.

44

Medical Emergencies in Pedodontics and their Management

1. **Which of the following is a cause of syncope?**
   A. Allergic reaction
   B. Hypertension
   C. Ischemia
   D. All of the above

2. **Symptoms of syncope are:**
   (i) Slow and weak pulse
   (ii) Decreased blood pressure
   (iii) Increased respiratory rate
   (iv) Rash on face
   A. (i) and (ii) only
   B. (i) and (iii) only
   C. (i), (ii) and (iii) only
   D. (i), (ii), (iii) and (iv)

3. **For a patient with non-cyanotic congenital heart disease, in dental clinic:**
   A. Medical consultation is done
   B. Sedative premedication is given
   C. Preoperative antibiotic prophylaxis is done
   D. All of the above

4. **The optimum time for dental treatment of a patient suffering from chronic renal failure is:**
   A. One day after dialysis
   B. One week after dialysis
   C. 15 days after dialysis
   D. One month after dialysis

Answers

1.C. Syncope is a temporary loss of consciousness due to generalized cerebral ischemia.

2.C. Other symptoms include cold clammy skin, dilated pupils, eyes rolled upwards and loss of consciousness.

3.D. In acyanotic heart disease due to a cardiac effect blood is shunted from left to right. The group mainly includes ventricular and atrial septal defects and defects that cause obstruction.

4.A. In case patient is on dialysis, treatment is done one day after dialysis, when heparin is no longer a factor in hemostasis (half-life:4 hours).

45

Management of Handicapped Children

1. **Children with Down's syndrome suffer from:**
   A. Mental deficiency
   B. Growth retardation
   C. Destructive periodontal diseases
   D. All of the above

2. **Hemophilia is transmitted from:**
   A. Male to male **B.** Female to female
   C. Female to male **D.** Male to female

3. **Hemophilia A is caused by deficiency of:**
   A. Factor V **B.** Factor VI
   C. Factor VII **D.** Factor VIII

4. **Christmas disease is caused by deficiency of:**
   A. Factor VIII **B.** Factor IX
   C. Factor X **D.** Factor V

5. **Mentally retarded children have IQ:**
   A. Below 50 **B.** Below 70
   C. Below 90 **D.** Below 100

6. **A child has a history of generalized growth failure ("failure to thrive") during the first six months of his life. Which of the following dental sequela is likely in this child?**
   A. Enamel hypoplasia **B.** Retrusive midface
   C. Retrusive mandible **D.** Small permanent teeth

7. **Which of the following best describes the usual behavioral characteristics of a child who has Down's syndrome?**
   A. Crying and stubbornness
   B. Hyperactive and disoriented
   C. Smiling, affectionate and easily distracted
   D. Fearful and unresponsive to verbal communication

Answers

1.D. Systemic factors which contribute are poor circulation , decreased humoral, response general physical deterioration and genetic influences.

2.C. Factor VIII is the most common of hemophilia and is inherited as an X-linked recessive trait. Therefore, males are affected and females are carriers. It is not transmitted from male to male.

3.D. Hemophilia B or Christmas disease is caused by a deficiency in factor IX.

4.B. Factor IX is also known as plasma thromoboplastin antecedent.

5.B. Mental retardation is defined as "Significantly subaverage intellectual functioning existing concurrently with deficits in adaptive behaviour and manifested during developmental period."

6.A. A child having a history of generalized growth failure during the first 6 months of his life suffer from enamel hypoplasia.

7.C. Down's syndrome is also known as Trisorny 21 syndrome. Patients have several aberrant features such as reduced height, small head with prominent forehead, short neck, short hands, etc.

46

Oral Manifestations of Systemic Diseases in Children and their Management

1. **Characteristic feature of hypopituitarism is:**
   A. Delayed eruption of dentition
   B. Primary teeth do not resorb
   C. Permanent teeth do not erupt
   D. All of the above

2. **Enamel hypoplasia is caused by:**
   A. Hypoparathyroidism
   B. Chronic renal disease
   C. Intestinal malabsorption syndrome
   D. All of the above

3. **Common age group of rheumatic heart fever affected patient is:**
   A. 0 to 6 years   B. 6 to 15 years
   C. 15 to 25 years   D. 20 to 30 years

4. **In patients suffering from cardiac disease, oral infection may lead to:**
   A. Infectious mononucleosis
   B. Lymphoma
   C. Subacute bacterial endocarditis
   D. Exacerbation of disease

5. **Oral manifestations of diabetic mellitus are:**
   A. Oral candidiasis
   B. Oral ulcerations
   C. Increased severity of periodontitis and bone loss
   D. All of the above

6. **Reduced vertical height of mandible and open bite is the oral manifestation of:**
   A. Hypothyroidism
   B. Hypopituitarism
   C. Hypoparathyroidism
   D. Hyperthyroidism

7. **'Chvostek's sign' is the oral manifestation of:**
   A. Hypothyroidism
   B. Hypopituitarism
   C. Hypoparathyroidism
   D. Hyperthyroidism

8. **Heat intolerance, loss of weight despite increased appetite, exophthalmos, widening of palpebral fissures, lid-lag are the signs and symptoms of:**
   A. Hypothyroidism
   B. Hyperpituitarism
   C. Hyperparathyroidism
   D. Hyperthyroidism

9. **Radiographically, "ground glass" appearance of jaws is commonly seen in:**
   A. Hyperpituitarism
   B. Hyperthyroidism
   C. Hypercalcemia
   D. Hypoparathyroidism

10. **Micrognathia, decreased lower facial height and obtuse gonial angle are most commonly seen in:**
    A. Systemic lupus erythematosus
    B. Juvenile rheumatoid arthritis
    C. Dermatomyositis
    D. Scleroderma

11. **Strawberry tongue is most commonly found in:**
    A. Scarlet fever
    B. Acute necrotizing ulcerative gingivitis
    C. Recurrent aphthous stomatitis
    D. Congenital syphilis

12. **The pseudomembranous papilla and punched-out shaped erosions are found in:**
    A. Scarlet fever
    B. ANUG
    C. Congenital syphilis
    D. Recurrent aphthous stomatitis

13. **The notched incisors and mulberry molars are most commonly found in:**
    - **A.** Scarlet fever
    - **B.** ANUG
    - **C.** Congenital syphilis
    - **D.** Recurrent aphthous stomatitis

14. **Oral lesion(s) associated with HIV infection in a child is:**
    - **A.** Oral candidiasis
    - **B.** Parotid swelling
    - **C.** Hairy leukoplakia
    - **D.** All of the above

15. **'World AIDS Day' is observed on:**
    - **A.** 1st November
    - **B.** 15th November
    - **C.** 1st December
    - **D.** 15th December

16. **Which of the following is not a major sign and symptom of AIDS?**
    - **A.** Weight loss more than 10% of body weight in one month
    - **B.** Chronic diarrhea for more than a month
    - **C.** Prolonged fever for more than a month
    - **D.** Persistent cough for more than a month

17. **Hutchinson's triad is found in:**
    - **A.** Congenital syphilis
    - **B.** ANUG
    - **C.** Juvenile rheumatoid arthritis
    - **D.** Scarlet fever

Answers

1.D. Vertical height of the mandible is reduced resulting in open bite, immature facial patterns, reduced intermaxillary space and crowding of the teeth.

2.D. In chronic renal failure, hypoplasia with a classic appearance of regular incremental defects affecting teeth in the appositional of development has been reported.

3.B. Rheumatic heart fever is a very serious inflammatory disease that occurs as a delayed sequela to pharyngeal infections with group A streptococci.

4.C. Subacute bacterial endocarditis usually develops in persons with pre-existing congenital cardiac disease or rheumatic valvular lesions.

5.D. Diabetes mellitus is a group of symptoms and findings, with the basic underlying problem of glucose intolerance.

6.B. Hypopituitarism results from anterior pituatary insufficiency. It is either idiopathic or secondary to pituatory or hypothalamic diseases.

7.C. In Chvostek's sign, a sharp tap in front of the ear over the facial nerve causes twitching of facial muscles around the mouth.

8.D. Hyperthyroidism is the hyperfunction of thyroid gland .It is more common in females between the ages of 12 and 14 years.

9.C. Ground glass appearance of jaws is also seen in chronic renal failure.

10.B. Juvenile rheumatoid arthritis is a disease or group of diseases characterized by chronic deforming arthritis.

11.A. The papillae become reddened and edematous and project through the white coat producing so called strawberry tongue.

12.B. Acute necrotizing ulcerative gingivitis is a fusospirochetal infection and referred to as trench mouth.

13.C. The Hutchinson triad is pathognomonic of congenital syphilis.

14.D. Oral candidiasis is characterized as a white plaque on the dorsum of the tongue in children.

15.C. All dental professionals must recognize HIV infected patients. These innocent sufferers form a special group with special needs and precautions. Therefore, all possible efforts must be made to deliver quality dental services to them.

16.D. WHO has defined AIDS as the existence of two major signs associated with atleast one minor sign, in the absence of known secondary causes of immunosuppression.

17.A. Congenital syphilis is caused by *Treponema pallidum*, transmitted by an infected mother.

47

Infection Control and AIDS

1. **Root canal instruments should be sterilized by:**
   A. Moist heat
   B. Dry heat
   C. Glass bead sterilizer
   D. Disinfectants

2. **Autoclaving is done at:**
   A. 120°C for 30 min
   B. 150°C for 20 min
   C. 150°C for 30 min
   D. 180°C for 15 min

3. **The international and Govt. of India's color coding for infectious wastes is:**
   A. Red
   B. Black
   C. Yellow
   D. Blue

Answers

1.C. Root canal instrument and burs should be washed with alcohol and than sterilized at a temperature of 210 to 230°C for 30 seconds.

2.A. A ten minutes are enough for complete sterilization if high pressure vacuum autoclave is used at136°C at 22 lbs pressure.

3.C. The container should be prominently embossed with a sticker or labeled "biohazard". It will be preferable if these boxes should be made unpilferable by reducing the size of the opening.

48

LASERs in Pedodontics

1. **Which of the following is not a use of laser in Pedodontics?**
   A. Endodontic treatment
   B. Analgesic effects and biostimulation
   C. Prevention of caries
   D. None

2. **Which of the following statements is true regarding lasers?**
   A. Reduce the enamel permeability
   B. Reduce the enamel solubility
   C. Form an acid resistant superficial sealed layer of dentin
   D. All of the above

Answers

1.D. LASER is the abbreviation of light (L), amplification (A), by stimulated (S), emission (E), of radiation (R).

2.D. Presence of surface defects like pits, fissures, cracks, etc act as pathways for the demineralizing agents like acids. Such surface defects are partially closed or fused by the application

49

High Speeds and Ultraspeeds in Pedodontics

1. **The high speed rotary instruments have the speed of:**
   - **A.** Up to 10,000 r.p.m
   - **B.** Up to 30,000 r.p.m.
   - **C.** 30,000 to 50,000 r.p.m.
   - **D.** 30,000 to 2,50,000 r.p.m.

2. **The disadvantage/s of slow speed is/are:**
   - **A.** Increased pain at the operating site
   - **B.** More pressure is required
   - **C.** Increased heat production and pulpal damage
   - **D.** All of the above

Answers

1.D. Conventional or low speed rotary instruments have the speed below 30,000 rpm.

2.D. Slow speed also causes increased vibration and slow cutting.

50

Epidemiology of Dental Diseases in Children in India

1. Occurrence of new cases in a defined population during a specified period is known as:

A. Incidence
B. Prevalence
C. Epidemic
D. Endemic

2. Incidence rate is calculated as:

$$\frac{\text{Number of new cases of the specific disease during a given year in a population}}{\text{Total number of population at risk in that year}} \times \ldots\ldots$$

A. 10
B. 100
C. 1000
D. 10,000

3. Point prevalence is calculated as:

$$\frac{\text{Total number of existing (new and old) cases of a specified disease during a given period of time}}{\text{Estimated population at that same point of time}} \ldots\ldots$$

A. 10
B. 100
C. 1000
D. 10,000

4. Epidemiological tetrad consists of:

A. Etiological agent, host, time period, diet
B. Etiological agent, host, environment, time period
C. Physical agent (heat, cold) , time period, host, environment
D. Duration, agent, time period, host

Answers

1.A. As a health status indicator the incidence rate is useful to: (a) prevent and control disease, (b) ascertain etiology and pathogenesis, and (c) determine the efficacy of preventive and therapeutic measures .

2.D. Prevalence means the total number of cases (new and old) of a specific disease in existence in a given population at a particular period of time or at a point of time.

3.B. When only the prevalence rate is used without any further clarification, it is taken to mean point prevalence. It can be specified for age, sex and other relevant factors.

4.B. Environment is the total sum of all the external influences and conditions affecting the life and development of an organism, human behavior and society.

51

Miscellaneous

All India PGDEE 2004

1. **Which of the following is the most recommended endodontic obturating material for deciduous teeth?**
   A. KR-1 paste
   B. ZOE
   C. $Ca(OH)_2$ paste
   D. Maisto's paste

2. **The current recommendation for breast-feeding is that:**
   A. Exclusive breast-feeding should be continued till 6 months of age followed by supplementation with additional foods.
   B. Exclusive breast-feeding should be continued till 4 months of age followed by supplementation with additional foods.
   C. Colostrum is the most suitable food for a new born baby but it is best avoided in first 2 days
   D. The baby should be allowed to breast-feed till one year of age.

3. **Into how many segments the infant's gum pad is divided:**
   A. Two in each quadrant
   B. Three in each quadrant
   C. Two in each jaw
   D. Five in each quadrant

4. **Which statement best describes tooth development during eruption:**
   A. The crown pierces the alveolar crest when b root is complete
   B. The crown reaches the occlusal plane when b root is complete
   C. The crown pierces the alveolar crest when ¾ of root is complete
   D. The crown does not emerge in the oral cavity until root formation is complete

5. Patients with Down's Syndrome normally have:

A. IQ score above 80
B. Brachycephalic skull
C. Stiff muscles
D. All of the above

6. What is the latest name of multiple caries in children involving most of the teeth?

A. Rampant caries
B. Maternally derived *Strepotoccus mutans* disease
C. Early childhood caries
D. Early childhood syndrome

7. Which of the following antibiotic prescribed in case of juvenile periodontitis?

A. Tetracycline
B. Erythromycine
C. Sulfadiazine
D. Cephalexin

Answers

1.A. KR-1 or Walkoff's paste is resorbable endodontic sealing paste consisting of Iodo form 60 parts in a complex mixture of 40 parts of camphor 49% parachloraphenal 45% and menthol 6%.

2.A. Mother's milk remains the ideal food for a child despite the cariogenic potential. By way of colostrums, it provides a natural transfer of immunoglobulins.

3.D. Gum pads is divided by transverse grooves into ten segments (five in each quadrant), each corresponding to a deciduous tooth sac and is at first papillomatous.

4.A. The time interval between crown completion and beginning of eruption until the tooth is in full occlusion is approximately 3 to 5 years for permanent teeth .

5.B. Children with Down's syndrome suffer from rapid destructive periodontal diseases related to tooth morphology bruxism, malocclusion and poor oral hygiene .

6.A. According to Massler, definition of rampant dental caries is "a suddenly appearing ,widespread , rapidly burrowing type of caries, resulting in early involvement of the pulp and affecting those teeth usually regarded as immune to ordinary decay." Rampant caries involves atleast ten new teeth surfaces with new lesions per year.

7.A. Juvenile periodontitis can be defined as the general term used to include a degenerative, noninflammatory destruction of the periodontium originating in one or more of the periodontal structures.

All India PGDEE 2005

1. **Mouth guards to prevent accidents to teeth are most practical for:**
   A. All children
   B. All persons engaged in contact sports
   C. Automobile passengers
   D. Persons on organized athletic team

2. **As age advances, the human profile generally:**
   A. Remain the same
   B. Increases in convexity
   C. Decreases in convexity
   D. Decreases in concavity

3. **Class II cavity preparation for amalgam restoration in deciduous teeth requires:**
   A. More buccolingual extension
   B. More mesiodistal extension
   C. More gingival
   D. More cervical

4. **Hand over mouth technique was first described by:**
   A. Dr. Evangeline Jordan **B.** Addelson and Goldfried
   C. Dr. G.V. Black **D.** Dr. Goldman

5. **Oral screen:**
   A. Causes the child to breathe through the nose
   B. Prevents passage of air through mouth
   C. Prevents passage of air through nares
   D. Allows the passage of air through mouth and nose

6. **Ormocers are:**
   A. Organically modified composites
   B. Inorganically modified composites
   C. Organically modified Glass Inomer cement
   D. Inorganically modified Glass Inomer cement

7. **Speech retardation may be considered if the child does not talk by:**
   A. 12 months **B.** 18 months
   C. 24 months **D.** 36 months

8. By what age does the startle and grasp reflex disappear?

A. 1 year
B. 1 ½ years
C. 2 years
D. 3 years

9. Who proposed the operant conditioning theory of child psychology:

A. Pavlov
B. Skinner
C. Jean Piaget
D. Sigmond Freud

10. According to the Freudian psychosexual stages of development the stage which corresponds with development of mixed dentition and character formation is:

A. Concrete operational
B. Latency
C. Phallic
D. Genital

11. Caries activity test that gives a quantitative determination of the acidogenic microorganism in the oral cavity:

A. Fosdick test
B. Synder test
C. Alban's test
D. Salivary Reductase test

12. Which position is the most important in diagnosis of anterior or posterior crossbite?

A. Habitual position
B. Lateral shift
C. Maximum intercuspation
D. The point of first contact at centric relation

Answers

1.B. The accidents to teeth and jaw can be prevented or significantly reduced by use of mouth guards by athletes who are engaged in contact sports.

2.C. At birth mandible is retrognathic to the maxilla giving the face convex appearance. Later on rapid growth of mandible decreases the convexity of profile.

3.A. As the primary molars have broad contact area and we have to put the cavity wall in self cleansing area so more of the buccolingual extension is required.

4.A. Hand over mouth technique was described by Evangeline Jordan for dealing with very uncooperative child. Here hand is placed over the child's mouth and speaking quietly into his ear that hand will only be removed as he/ she stops crying. When child responds and stops crying the hand is immediately removed.

5.A. Oral (vestibular) screen is used to stop mouth breathing habit. By this air is prevented from entering the oral cavity and child is forced to breath through nose.

6.B. Ormocers are organically modified composites while ceramic optimized composite are called as ceromers.

7.C. For language to develop normal, child auditory and visual systems must be normal because blind and deaf children have delayed language development.

8.C. Startle reflex is generally due to sudden noise and in grasp reflex when baby's palm is stimulated the hand closes. Both the reflexes disappear at the age of 2 year.

9.B. Operant conditioning theory of child psychology was given by Skinner while Pavlov gave the classical conditioning theory.

10.B. Time duration of phallic stage is 3 to 5 years while latency ranges from 10 to 11 year, which is the time for mixed dentition.

11.A. Snyder and Alban are qualitative methods on the basis of salivary acid uric organisms. Reductase test is also qualitative method but it shows about total salivary organism. Fosdick test is quantitative method and measures the buffering capacity of total salivary organism.

12.C. Anterior or posterior crossbites are diagnosed when both the dental arches are brought into maximum intercuspation.

All India PGDEE 2006

1. **The partial pulpotomy technique was advocated by:**
   A. Bowen in 1974
   B. Clarke in 1976
   C. Cvek in 1978
   D. Willet in 1980

2. **Distal shoe was first advocated by whom in 1929?**
   A. Wilson
   B. Willet
   C. Wilhem
   D. Roche

3. **Incipient or recurrent caries can be detected before they are visible on the radiograph by:**
   A. Visible light
   B. Ultrasonic light
   C. Fibreoptic transillumination
   D. Digital imaging fibreoptic transillumination

4. **Stainless steel crowns are contraindicated in:**
   A. Medically compromised patient (VSD. ASD)
   B. After endodontic therapy
   C. Rampant caries
   D. Amelogenesis imperfecta

Answers

1.C. In young teeth only superficial pulp from the pulp chamber is removed in the partial pulpotomy.

2.B. The Willett distal guiding shoe has been a commonly placed space maintainer in case of unilateral loss of deciduous second molar. It was introduced in 1929 and is designed to be inserted into the soft tissues and bony alveolus to guide the erupting permanent molar.

3.D. Early decalcification can be detected by Digital imaging fibreoptic transillumination.

4.A. Stainless steel crowns are contraindicated in

i. Anterior teeth where esthetics is required.

ii. Medically compromised patient.